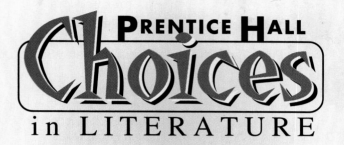

PRENTICE HALL
Choices
in LITERATURE

The Adventure of Me
Joining Hands
It's Up to You
Conflict and Resolution
The World of "What if . . . ?"

The Me You See
Where Paths Meet
Deciding What's Right
You Are the Solution
Communication Explosion

Myself, My World
American Tapestry
Justice for All
Making a Difference
Charting Your Own Course

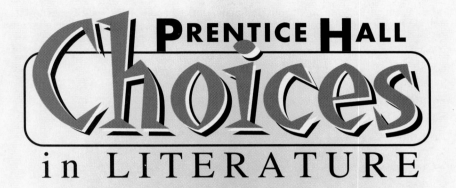

PRENTICE HALL
Choices
in LITERATURE

Deciding What's Right

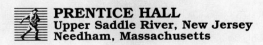

PRENTICE HALL
Upper Saddle River, New Jersey
Needham, Massachusetts

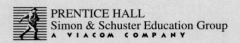

PRENTICE HALL
Simon & Schuster Education Group
A VIACOM COMPANY

Staff Credits for Prentice Hall Choices in Literature

(In Alphabetical Order)

Advertising and Promotion: Carol Leslie, Alfonso Manosalvas, Rip Odell

Business Office: Emily Heins

Design: Laura Bird, Eric Dawson, Jim O'Shea, Carol Richman, AnnMarie Roselli, Gerry Schrenk

Editorial: Ellen Bowler, Megan Chill, Barbara W. Coe, Elisa Mui Eiger, Philip Fried, Rebecca Z. Graziano, Douglas McCollum

Manufacturing and Inventory Planning: Katherine Clarke, Rhett Conklin, Matt McCabe

Marketing: Jean Faillace, Mollie Ledwith

Media Resources: Libby Forsyth, Maureen Raymond

National Language Arts Consultants: Kathy Lewis, Karen Massey, Craig A. McGhee, Vennisa Travers, Gail Witt

Permissions: Doris Robinson

Pre-press Production: Carol Barbara, Kathryn Dix, Marie McNamara, Annette Simmons

Production: Margaret Antonini, Christina Burghard, Greg Myers, Marilyn Stearns, Cleasta Wilburn

Sales: Ellen Backstrom

Acknowledgments

Grateful acknowledgment is made to the following for permission to reprint copyrighted material:

Miriam Altschuler Literary Agency as agent for Walter Dean Myers
"The Treasure of Lemon Brown" by Walter Dean Myers from *Boy's Life Magazine,* March 1983. Copyright © 1983 by Walter Dean Myers. Reprinted by permission of Miriam Altschuler Agency as agent for the author.

Arte Público Press
"Believe in Yourself" by Sandra María Esteves is reprinted with permission from the publisher of *Bluestown Mockingbird Mambo* (Houston: Arte Público Press-University of Houston, 1990). "Immigrants" from *Borders* by Pat Mora is reprinted from *Borders* (Houston: Arte Público Press-University of Houston, 1986).

Curtis Brown Ltd.
The Boy Who Drew Sheep by Anne Rockwell first appeared in *The Boy Who Drew Sheep* published by Atheneum. Copyright © 1973 by Anne Rockwell. Reprinted by permission of Curtis Brown Ltd.

Eric Chock
"The Bait" by Eric Chock reprinted from *Last Days Here* (Bamboo Ridge Press, 1990). Copyright © 1989 Eric Chock. Reprinted by permission of the author.

Dell Books, a division of Bantam Doubleday Dell Publishing Group, Inc.
"The Tail" by Joyce Hansen, copyright © 1992 by Joyce Hansen, from *Funny You Should Ask* by David Gale, Editor. Used by permission of Dell Books, a division of Bantam Doubleday Dell Publishing Group, Inc.

(Continued on page H181.)

Deciding What's Right

Contents

Looking at Literary Forms: Folk Tales

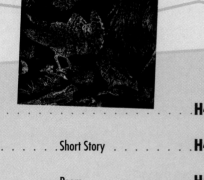

WHAT IS MY RESPONSIBILITY TO OTHERS?

Looking at Literary Forms: Drama

WHAT MATTERS MOST? **H123**

About This Program

What makes reading exciting?

Reading is a great way to learn more about the world and about yourself. Reading gives you the chance to make a movie in your mind and experience adventures you might never be able to actually live. Words can take you to faraway lands, tell you about important discoveries and courageous people, make you laugh and cry, or let you look at your world in a new way.

How will reading pay off in your future?

Beyond being entertaining, reading is important. As you learn more, you increase your choices in life. The skills and strategies you practice today will help you to become a life-long learner—someone who has questions, reads to answer them, and develops more questions!

How will this book help you get more out of what you read?

This book and your teacher will help you become a better reader. The selections included will grab your attention and help you practice specific skills valuable to the reading process.

Questions and activities at the beginning of selections will help you relate the reading to your own life; questions at the end will help you expand on what you learned. Activities and projects throughout the book will help you generate and explore new pathways of learning.

What features make this book a great learning tool?

* **Artwork to Spark Your Interest** Fine art, student art, photography, and maps can give you clues about the writing and direct the way you read.

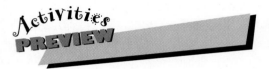

* **Exciting Activities to Get You Into the Selection** A preview page for each selection asks a question to get you thinking. Stop and consider your own responses to this question. Talk with classmates to get their ideas. As you read, you may find your own opinions changing. Reading can do that, too.

 The **Reach Into Your Background** feature will always give you ideas for connecting the selection to your own experience. In many cases, you may know more than you think you do. Try the activities in this section for a jump start before you read. Don't expect to be in your seats all the time! You'll learn more about your ideas by role-playing, debating, and sharing what you know with others.

* **Useful Strategies to Help You Through the Selection** This program will teach you essential techniques for getting more out of your reading.

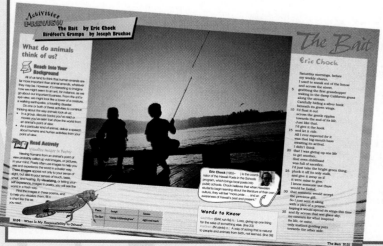

In **Read Actively** you'll find hands-on approaches to getting more out of what you read. Here's your chance to practice the skills that will bring you reading success. You'll learn to make inferences, gather evidence, set a purpose for reading, and much more. Once you've learned these skills, you can use them in all the reading that you do . . . and you'll get more out of your reading.

Some of the strategies you'll learn include:

Identifying Problems

Making Judgments

Asking Questions

Visualizing Characters

Setting a Purpose for Reading

Recognizing a Sequence of Events

Connecting Nonfiction to Your Own Experience

Responding to Literature

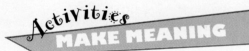

MAKE MEANING

• Thought-Provoking Activities to Generate New Ideas Following each selection, you'll have the chance to explore your own ideas and learn more about what you read.

Explore Your Reading takes you into, through, and beyond the actual selection to help you investigate the writing and its ideas more closely.

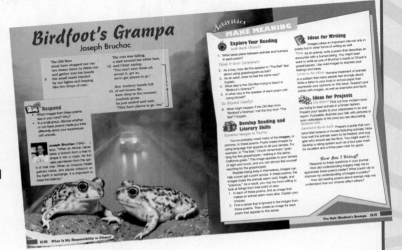

Develop Reading and Literary Skills expands your knowledge of literary forms, terms, and techniques. Following up on the Read Actively activities and strategies, you will learn more about how writing communicates.

Ideas for Writing and **Ideas for Projects** offer you the chance to create your own answers to your own questions. How does the selection relate to you? Where can you learn more? What cross-curricular connections can you make? These ideas features help you try things out yourself.

Enjoy this book!

All the features of this program fit together to develop your interest, skills, and, ultimately, your ability to learn.

Have fun with the time you spend with this book. Look at the art, plan for unit level projects, look for connections between selections. Pay attention to your own questions—finding the answers to those may be the most rewarding of all.

Deciding What's Right

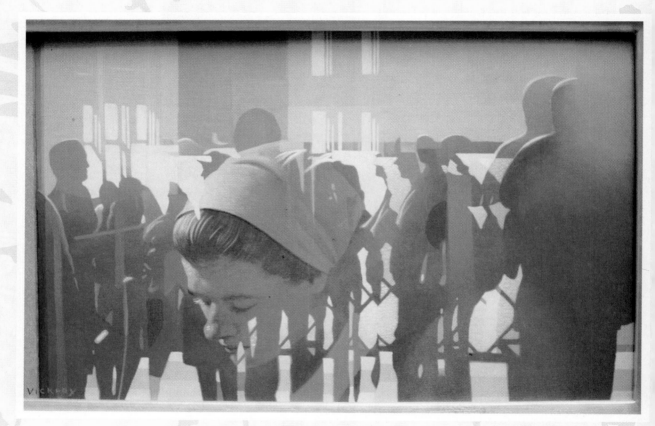

Untitled Robert Vickrey ©1996 Robert Vickrey, Licensed by VAGA, New York, New York

"We know what a person thinks not when he tells us what he thinks, but by his actions." — **Isaac Bashevis Singer**

Get the Picture

Think about what Isaac Bashevis Singer is telling you as you look at the picture. You too have had to make decisions and deal with what is right and what is wrong. How do you make that kind of decision? In answering this question, you may ask yourself questions like these:

- ## What Are My Choices?
- ## What Is My Responsibility to Others?
- ## What Matters Most?

The authors in this unit have thought about these questions and their answers might give you new insights to add to your own ideas. Keep a journal for "Deciding What's Right." As you read the selections in this unit, you can use your journal to write your own questions, answer them, and reflect on what you've read and learned.

Activities
In a Group With several classmates, discuss the decision-making strategies people your age use each day. Your group might list the kinds of decisions you make, the people who give you advice, how much time you take to decide, and the steps you take when you face an important decision.

Activities
On Your Own Use the first page of your journal to make a cluster diagram that shows what matters most to you. Write your name in the center of the page. Then draw lines out from your name to show people, places, things, and ideas that have special meaning for you.

Project Preview . . . .

You can also respond to questions about what is right by working on exciting projects. Preview the following projects and choose one that you might like to do. For more details, see page H162.

- **Career Day Fair**

- **Choices-and-Consequences Cartoons**

- **Way-to-Go Awards**

- **Public Service Television Campaign**

- **Multimedia Presentation: What Matters Most**

- **Illustrated Book of What Matters**

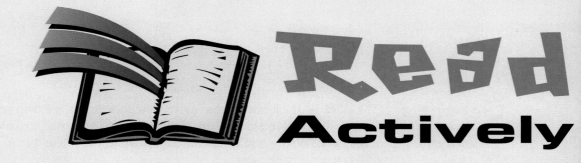

Read Actively

How does my reading relate to my world?

How can I get more from what I read?

The answer to questions like these is to be an active reader, an *involved* reader. As an active reader, you are in charge of the reading situation!

The following strategies tell how to think as an active reader. You don't need to use all of these strategies all of the time. Feel free to choose the ones that work best in each reading situation.

BEFORE YOU READ

PREVIEW

What do the title and the pictures suggest? What will the selection say about "Deciding What's Right"?

GIVE YOURSELF A PURPOSE

What is the author communicating?
What will you learn about the theme?
How will the selection relate to your life?

REACH INTO YOUR BACKGROUND

What do you know already?

WHiLE yOU READ

AFTER yOU READ

PREDICT

What do you think will happen? Why?
You can change your mind as you read along.

ASK QUESTIONS

What's happening? Why do the characters
do what they do? Why does the author give
you certain details or use a particular word?
Your questions help you gather evidence
and make inferences.

VISUALIZE

What would these events and characters
look like in a movie? How would the writer's
descriptions look in a photograph?

CONNECT

Are characters like you or someone you know?
What would you do in a similar situation?

RESPOND

Talk about what you've read.
What did you think?

ASSESS YOURSELF

How did you do? Were your predictions
on target? Did you find answers to
your questions?

FOLLOW UP

Show what you know. Get involved!
Do a project. Keep learning.

The model that begins on the next page
shows Barry Johnson's thoughts while actively
reading "The Princess and the Tin Box."

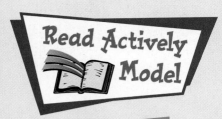
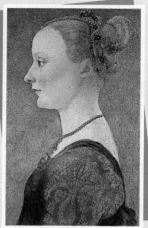

Portrait Of A Young Lady, c. 1470
Piero del Pollaiuolo
Metropolitan Museum of Art

I think that when the princess gets old enough, her father will make her marry a rich or handsome guy. [Predict]

Hi! My name is Barry Johnson and I attend Ralph Bunch Middle School in Atlanta, Georgia. I expected this fairy tale to have a moral that would teach me a valuable lesson. As I read, I wrote the notes you see in the margins.

Barry Johnson

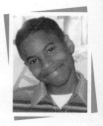

The Princess and the Tin Box

James Thurber

Once upon a time, in a far country, there lived a king whose daughter was the prettiest princess in the world. Her eyes were like the cornflower, her hair was sweeter than the hyacinth, and her throat made the swan look dusty.

From the time she was a year old, the princess had been showered with presents. Her nursery looked like Cartier's[1] window. Her toys were all made of gold or platinum or diamonds or emeralds. She was not permitted to have wooden blocks or china dolls or rubber dogs or linen books, because such materials were considered cheap for the daughter of a king.

When she was seven, she was allowed to attend the wedding of her bother and throw real pearls at the bride instead of rice. Only the nightingale, with his lyre[2] of gold, was permitted to sing for the princess. The common blackbird, with his boxwood flute, was kept out of the palace grounds. She walked in silver-and-samite slippers to a sapphire-and-topaz bathroom and slept in an ivory bed inlaid with rubies.

On the day the princess was eighteen, the king sent a royal ambassador to the courts of five neighboring kingdoms to announce that he would give his daughter's hand in marriage to the prince who brought her the gift she liked most.

The first prince to arrive at the palace rode a swift white stallion and laid at the feet of the princess an enormous apple made of solid gold which he had taken from a dragon who had guarded it for a thousand years. It was placed on a long ebony table set up to hold the gifts of the princess's suitors. The second prince, who came on a gray charger, brought her a nightingale made of a thousand diamonds, and it was placed beside the golden apple. The third prince, riding on a black horse, carried a great jewel box made of platinum and sapphires, and it was placed next to the diamond nightingale. The fourth prince, astride a fiery yellow horse, gave the princess a gigantic heart

You can tell this is a fairy tale. The people I know would never give a girl a golden apple. [Connect]

1. **Cartier's:** A well-known upscale jewelry store.
2. **lyre** (LĪR) *n.*: Harp.

made of rubies and pierced by an emerald arrow. It was placed next to the platinum-and-sapphire jewel box.

Now the fifth prince was the strongest and handsomest of all the five suitors, but he was the son of a poor king whose realm had been overrun by mice and locusts and wizards and mining engineers so that there was nothing much of value left in it. He came plodding up to the palace of the princess on a plow horse and he brought her a small tin box filled with mica and feldspar and hornblende[3] which he had picked up on the way.

The other princes roared with disdainful laughter when they saw the tawdry gift the fifth prince had brought to the princess. But she examined it with great interest and squealed with delight, for all her life she had been glutted with precious stones and priceless metals, but she had never seen tin before or mica or feldspar or hornblende. The tin box was placed next to the ruby heart pierced with an emerald arrow.

"Now," the king said to his daughter, "you must select the gift you like best and marry the prince that brought it."

The princess smiled and walked up to the table and picked up the present she liked the most. It was the platinum-and-sapphire jewel box, the gift of the third prince.

"The way I figure it," she said, "is this. It is a very large and expensive box, and when I am married, I will meet many admirers who will give me the precious gems with which to fill it to the top. Therefore, it is the most valuable of all the gifts my suitors have brought me and I like it the best."

The princess married the third prince that very day in the midst of great merriment and high revelry. More than a hundred thousand pearls were thrown at her and she loved it.

Moral: All those who thought the princess was going to select the tin box filled with worthless stones instead of one of the other gifts will kindly stay after class and write one hundred times on the blackboard, "I would rather have a hunk of aluminum silicate than a diamond necklace."

---

3. mica (MĪ kuh), **feldspar** (FELD spahr), **hornblende** (HAWRN blend) *ns.*: Common minerals found in rocks.

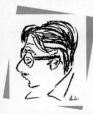

James Thurber (1894–1961) is remembered as a humorist whose stories poked fun at the modern world. Even the titles of his works show his unique form of comedy. One collection of stories is called *The Middle-Aged Man on the Flying Trapeze.*

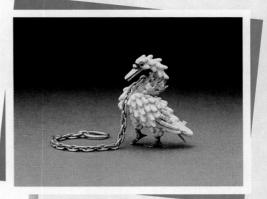

The Dunstable Swan made by a London goldsmith, c.1400 British Museum

I think a princess should have a man that is good to her no matter how rich or handsome he is. [Respond]

I think she'll choose the tin box. She should pick the man that will respect and love her. [Predict]

My prediction was off by a mile! [Check prediction]

Respond

- If you had been the princess, what choice would you have made?
- In a small group, discuss the ending of the fairy tale. What did you find surprising about it and why?

At left: *James Thurber self-portrait*
James Thurber
The Granger Collection, New York

Activities
MAKE MEANING

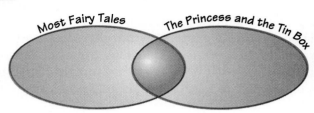

Explore Your Reading

Look Back (Recall)

1. What reasons does the princess give for her decision?

Think It Over (Interpret)

2. What do the princess's choice and her explanation of that choice tell you about her character? Explain.
3. What point is the writer making through this fairy tale and its moral? Explain.

Go Beyond (Apply)

4. The princess had to choose her husband based on a gift that he brought her. What information do you think people should use to decide whether or not to marry someone?

Develop Reading and Literary Skills

Understand Humor

Humor, writing meant to amuse and entertain, can make you aware of human nature even while you're laughing. In this selection, James Thurber makes fun of the traditional fairy tale to make a point about human nature.

For his comedy to be successful, Thurber relies on your knowledge and expectations of fairy tales. These traditional stories follow a set pattern so you may have expected a princess to choose the poor but handsome prince. However, this princess acts differently. She makes a practical, if selfish, decision when she chooses the rich prince with the jewelry box. This surprising switch makes the story funny and tells you something about people.

1. Complete a Venn diagram like the one on this page to show the similarities and differences between this mock fairy tale and traditional fairy tales. On the left side include events that happen in most fairy tales. On the right, include events that happen in this one. Where the circles overlap, jot down details the stories have in common.

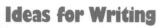

2. Use your diagram to state two other details that go against the reader's expectations of a fairy tale. Explain what makes these details humorous.

Ideas for Writing

Think about the traditional fairy tales you know and the lessons they teach.

Fairy Tale Create a humorous version of a traditional fairy tale. Use what you have learned from James Thurber to make your tale effective as well as amusing. Be sure that your fairy tale has a message for your readers, even if it is a comical one.

Comparison and Contrast Write an essay that compares and contrasts two characters in a traditional fairy tale. For example, you might tell about the differences and similarities between Cinderella's evil stepmother and her fairy godmother.

Ideas for Projects

Precious Gems Presentation Prepare a visual presentation, such as a large wall chart or a slide show about some of the gems that are mentioned in the story. Include the properties of the gems and metals and create colorful illustrations. [Science Link]

Readers Theater Find a fairy tale from another place or culture to present in a readers theater. To prepare for a dramatic reading of the story, divide and assign the narration of the story. Choose people to read the character's dialogue. Practice and present your readers theater to the rest of the class.

How Am I Doing?

Take a moment to answer these questions:
Which reading strategy helped me the most?
Which part of this fairy tale did I find funniest? Why?

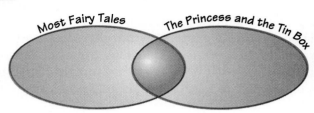

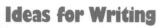

What Are My Choices?

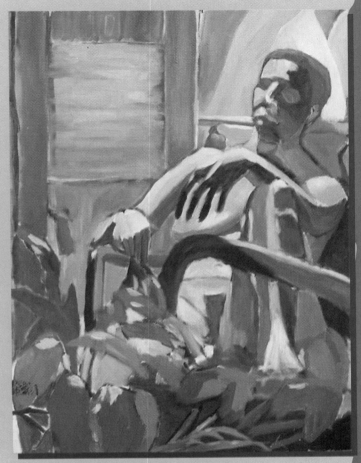

Student Art *Untitled* Guevera Soliman
Walt Whitman High School, Bethesda, Maryland

Coming Out of the Storm

Student Writing Summer Spisak, Mays Middle
Center for the Arts and Humanities, Miami, Florida

Destruction yet . . . togetherness
Desolation yet . . . consolation
New and old hearts mending . . . forgiveness
Quilt of life, sewn back together . . . whole again
Bravery and courage . . . kindness
Compassion and love . . . affection
Strength and stress, yet . . . friendship
Helpfulness . . . loving
      Peace

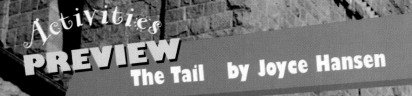

What is it like to look after someone younger?

Reach Into Your Background

At some time in your life, you've probably had to baby-sit. Maybe you've had to take care of a younger brother or sister or even a neighbor's child. Younger children can be fun to be around, but they can also be exhausting. At times, you may not even want the responsibility. Think back on your baby-sitting experiences by doing one or more of these activities with a small group:

- Discuss ways to keep a young child entertained and busy. Make a list of your best ideas.
- Imagine that you promised to baby-sit, but you got a more interesting offer from friends. Role-play the way you might treat the child you were asked to watch.

Read Actively
Identify Details That Create Suspense

If a child in your care were hurt, you would be worried. Stories can create a similar anxious feeling by using details that create **suspense,** a feeling of uncertainty about what will happen next. If you can recognize suspenseful details such as scary things people say or frightening objects, you will feel the suspense that involves you deeply in the story.

"The Tail" tells about a babysitting experience that is full of suspense. Make a chart like this one to discover how the tension builds. Look for scary objects, warning signs, and other clues to danger in the story.

Suspenseful Detail	Questions It Raises in Your Mind

The Tail

Joyce Hansen

◆

It began as the worst summer of my life. The evening before the first day of summer vacation, my mother broke the bad news to me. I was in the kitchen washing dishes and dreaming about the wonderful things my friends and I would be doing for two whole months—practicing for the annual double-dutch[1] contest, which we would definitely win; going to the roller skating rink, the swimming pool, the beach; and sleeping as late in the morning as I wanted to.

"Tasha," my ma broke into my happy thoughts, "your father and I decided that you're old enough now to take on certain responsibilities."

My heart came to a sudden halt. "Responsibilities?"

"Yes. You do know what that word means, don't you?"

---

1. **double-dutch:** A jump rope game in which two ropes are used at the same time.

I nodded, watching her dice an onion into small, perfect pieces.

"You're thirteen going on fourteen and your father and I decided that you're old enough to watch Junior this summer, because I'm going to start working again."

"Oh, no!" I broke the dish with a crash. "Not that, Mama." Junior is my seven-year-old brother and has been following me like a tail ever since he learned how to walk. And to make matters worse, there are no kids Junior's age on our block. Everyone is either older or younger than he is.

📖 **Read Actively**

Ask yourself what Tasha is thinking at this point.

I'd rather be in school than minding Junior all day. I could've cried.

"Natasha! There won't be a dish left in this house. You're not going to spend all summer ripping and roaring. You'll baby-sit Junior."

"But, Ma," I said, "it'll be miserable. That's not fair. All summer with Junior. I won't be able to play with my friends."

She wiped her hands on her apron. "Life ain't always fair."

I knew she'd say that.

Words to Know

annual (AN yoo uhl) *adj.*: Happening every year

"You'll still be able to play with your friends," she continued, "but Junior comes first. He is your responsibility. We're a family and we all have to help out."

◆

Mama went to work that next morning. Junior and I both stood by the door as she gave her last-minute instructions. Junior held her hand and stared up at her with an innocent look in his bright brown eyes, which everyone thought were so cute. Dimples decorated his round cheeks as he smiled and nodded at me every time Ma gave me an order. I knew he was just waiting for her to leave so he could torment me.

"Tasha, I'm depending on you. Don't leave the block."

"Yes, Ma."

"No company."

"Not even Naomi? She's my best friend."

"No company when your father and I are not home."

"Yes, Ma."

"Don't let Junior hike in the park."

"Yes, Ma."

"Make yourself and Junior a sandwich for lunch."

"Yes, Ma."

"I'll be calling you at twelve, so you'd better be in here fixing lunch. I don't want you all eating junk food all day long."

"Yes, Ma."

"Don't ignore Junior."

"Yes, Ma."

"Clean the breakfast dishes."

"Yes, Ma."

"Don't open the door to strangers."

"Yes, Ma."

Then she turned to Junior. "Now you, young man. You are to listen to your sister."

"Yes, Mommy," he sang out.

"Don't give her a hard time. Show me what a big boy you can be."

"Mommy, I'll do whatever Tasha say."

Words to Know

vow (VOW) *v.*: Promise; pledge

She kissed us both good-bye and left. I wanted to cry. A whole summer with Junior.

Junior turned to me and raised his right hand. "This is a vow of obedience." He looked up at the ceiling. "I promise to do whatever Tasha says."

"What do you know about vows?" I asked.

"I saw it on television. A man—"

"Shut up, Junior. I don't feel like hearing about some television show. It's too early in the morning."

I went into the kitchen to start cleaning, when the downstairs bell rang. "Answer the intercom,[2] Junior. If it's Naomi, tell her to wait for me on the stoop," I called out. I knew that it was Naomi, ready to start our big, fun summer. After a few minutes, the bell rang again.

"Junior!" I yelled. "Answer the intercom."

The bell rang again and I ran into the living room. Junior was sitting on the couch, looking at cartoons. "What's wrong with you? Why won't you answer the bell?"

He looked at me as if I were crazy. "You told me to shut up. I told you I'd do everything you say."

I pulled my hair. "See, you're bugging me already. Do something to help around here."

I pressed the intercom on the wall. "That you, Naomi?"

"Yeah."

"I'll be down in a minute. Wait for me out front."

"Okay."

I quickly washed the dishes. I couldn't believe how messed up my plans were. Suddenly there was a loud blast from the living room. I was so startled that I dropped a plate and it smashed to smithereens. Ma will kill me, I thought as I ran to the living room. It sounded like whole pieces of furniture were being sucked into the vacuum cleaner.

"Junior," I screamed over the racket, "you have it on too high."

He couldn't even hear me. I turned it off myself.

> 📖 **Read Actively**
>
> **Respond** to Junior's behavior. Do you know someone like him?

_____
2. **intercom** (IN tuhr kahm) *n.*: A communication system used in apartment buildings.

"What's wrong?"

"Ma vacuumed the living room last night. It doesn't need cleaning."

"You told me to do something to help," he whined.

I finished the dishes in a hurry so that I could leave the apartment before Junior bugged out again.

◆

I was so anxious to get outside that we ran down the four flights of stairs instead of waiting for the elevator. Junior clutched some comic books and his checkers game. He put his Mets baseball cap on backward as usual. Naomi sat on the stoop and Junior plopped right next to her like they were the best of friends.

"Hi, cutey." She smiled at him, turning his cap to the front of his head the way it was supposed to be. "What are we going to do today, Naomi?" he asked.

"Junior, you're not going to be in our faces all day," I snapped at him.

"Mama said you have to watch me. So I have to be in your face."

"You're baby-sitting, Tasha?" Naomi asked.

"Yeah." I told her the whole story.

"Aw, that's not so bad. At least you don't have to stay in the house. Junior will be good. Right, cutey?"

He grinned as she pinched his cheeks.

"See, you think he's cute because you don't have no pesty little brother or sister to watch," I grumbled.

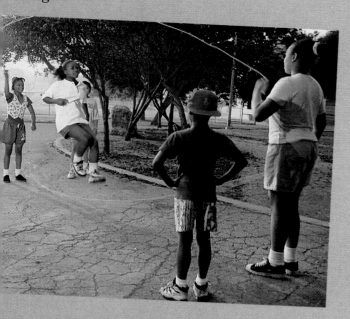

"You ready for double-dutch practice?" she asked. "Yvonne and Keisha are going to meet us in the playground."

"Mama said we have to stay on the block," Junior answered before I could even open my mouth.

"No one's talking to you, Junior." I pulled Naomi up off the stoop. "I promised my mother we'd stay on the block, but the playground is just across the street. I can see the block from there."

"It's still not the block," Junior mumbled as we raced across the street.

We always went over to the playground to jump rope. The playground was just by the entrance to the park. There was a lot of space for us to do our fancy steps. The park was like a big green mountain in the middle of Broadway.

I'd figure out a way to keep Junior from telling that we really didn't stay on the block. "Hey, Tasha, can I go inside the park and look for caves?" People said that if you went deep inside the park, there were caves that had been used centuries ago when Native Americans still lived in northern Manhattan.

"No, Ma said no hiking in the park."

"She said no leaving the block, too, and you left the block."

"Look how close we are to the block. I mean, we can even see it. You could get lost inside the park."

"I'm going to tell Ma you didn't stay on the block."

"Okay, me and Naomi will hike with you up to the Cloisters later." That's a museum that sits at the top of the park, overlooking the Hudson River. "Now read your comic books."

"Will you play checkers with me too?"

"You know I hate checkers. Leave me alone." I spotted Keisha and Yvonne walking into the playground. All of us wore shorts and sneakers.

Junior tagged behind me and Naomi as we went to meet them. "Remember you're supposed to be watching me," he said.

"How could I forget."

The playground was crowded. Swings were all taken and the older boys played stickball. Some little kids played in the sandboxes.

Keisha and Yvonne turned and Naomi and I jumped together, practicing a new routine. We were so good that some of the boys in the stickball game watched us. A few elderly people stopped to look at us too. We had an audience, so I really showed off—spinning and doing a lot of fancy footwork.

Suddenly Junior jumped in the ropes with us and people laughed and clapped.

"Junior!" I screamed. "Get out of here!"

"Remember, your job is to watch me." He grinned. My foot slipped and all three of us got tangled in the ropes and fell.

"Your feet are too big!" Junior yelled.

Everybody roared. I was too embarrassed. I tried to grab him, but he got away from me. "Get lost," I hollered after him as he ran toward the swings.

I tried to forget how stupid I must've looked and went back to the ropes. I don't know how long we'd been jumping when suddenly a little kid ran by us yelling, "There's a wild dog loose up there!" He pointed to the steps that led deep inside the park.

Read Actively

Ask yourself how this event builds suspense.

People had been saying for years that a pack of abandoned dogs who'd turned wild lived in the park, but no one ever really saw them.

We forgot about the kid and kept jumping. Then one of the boys our age who'd been playing stickball came over to us. "We're getting out of here," he said. "A big yellow dog with red eyes just bit a kid."

I took the rope from Yvonne. It was time for me and Naomi to turn. "That's ridiculous. Who ever heard of a yellow dog with red eyes?"

Naomi stopped turning. "Dogs look all kind of ways. Especially wild dogs. I'm leaving."

"Me too," Yvonne said.

Keisha was already gone. No one was in the swings or the sandboxes. I didn't even see the old men who usually sat on the benches. "Guess we'd better get out of here too," I said. Then I realized that I didn't see Junior anywhere.

"Junior!" I shouted.

"Maybe he went home," Naomi said.

We dashed across the street. Our block was empty. Yvonne ran ahead of us and didn't stop until she reached her stoop. When I got to my stoop I expected to see Junior there, but no Junior.

"Maybe he went upstairs," Naomi said.

"I have the key. He can't get in the house."

"Maybe he went to the candy store?"

"He doesn't have any money, I don't think. But let's look."

We ran around the corner to the candy store, but no Junior.

As we walked back to the block, I remembered something.

"Oh, no, Naomi, I told him to get lost. And that's just what he did."

"He's probably hiding from us somewhere. You know how he likes to tease." She looked around as we walked up our block. "He might be hiding and watching us right now looking for him." She peeped behind parked cars, in doorways, and even opened the lid of a trash can.

"Junior," I called. "Junior!"

No answer. Only the sounds of birds and cars, sirens and a distant radio. I looked at the empty stoop where Junior should have been sitting. A part of me was gone and I had to find it. And another part of me would be gone if my mother found out I'd lost Junior.

I ran back toward the playground and Naomi followed me. "He's got to be somewhere right around here," she panted.

I ran past the playground and into the park. "Tasha, you're not going in there, are you? The dog."

I didn't answer her and began climbing the stone steps that wound around and through the park. Naomi's eyes stretched all over her face and she grabbed my arm. "It's dangerous up here!"

I turned around. "If you're scared, don't come. Junior's my only baby brother. Dear God," I said out loud, "please let me find him. I will play any kind of game he wants. I'll never

Words to Know

gnawing (NAW ing) v.: Biting or wearing away bit by bit

mauled (MAWLD) v.: Attacked; handled roughly

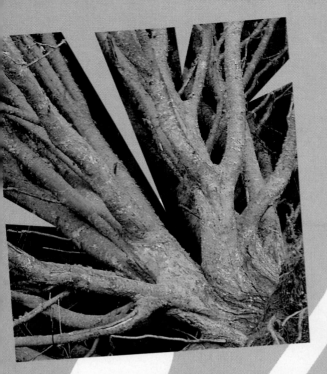

yell at him again. I promise never to be mean to him again in my life!"

Naomi breathed heavily behind me. "I don't think Junior would go this far by himself."

I stopped and caught my breath. The trees were thick and the city street sounds were far away now.

"I know Junior. He's somewhere up here making believe he's the king of this mountain. Hey, Junior," I called, "I was just kidding. Don't get lost." We heard a rustling in the bushes and grabbed each other. "Probably just a bird," I said, trying to sound brave.

As we climbed some more, I tried not to imagine a huge yellow dog with red eyes gnawing at my heels.

The steps turned a corner and ended. Naomi screamed and pointed up ahead. "What's that?"

I saw a big brown and gray monstrous thing with tentacles reaching toward the sky, jutting out of the curve in the path. I screamed and almost ran.

"What is that, Naomi?"

"I don't know."

"This is a park in the middle of Manhattan. It can't be a bear or anything." I screamed to the top of my lungs, "Junior!" Some birds flew out of a tree, but the thing never moved.

All Naomi could say was, "Dogs, Tasha."

I found a stick. "I'm going up. You wait here. If you hear growling and screaming, run and get some help." I couldn't believe how brave I was. Anyway, that thing, whatever it was, couldn't hurt me any more than my mother would if I didn't find Junior.

"You sure, Tasha?"

"No sense in both of us being mauled," I said.

I tipped lightly up the steps, holding the stick like a club. When I was a few feet away from the thing, I crumpled to the ground and laughed so hard that Naomi ran to me. "Naomi, look at what scared us."

She laughed too. "A dead tree trunk."

We both laughed until we cried. Then I saw one of Junior's comic books near a bush. I picked it up and started to cry. "See, he was here. And that animal probably tore him to pieces." Naomi patted my shaking shoulders.

Suddenly, there was an unbelievable growl. My legs turned to air as I flew down the steps. Naomi was ahead of me. Her two braids stuck out like propellers. My feet didn't even touch the ground. We screamed all the way down the steps. I tripped on the last step and was sprawled out on the ground. Two women passing by bent over me. "Child, are you hurt?" one of them asked.

📖 **Read Actively**
Predict what will happen next.

Then I heard a familiar laugh above me and looked up into Junior's dimpled face. He laughed so hard, he held his stomach with one hand. His checkers game was in the other. A little tan, mangy[3] dog stood next to him, wagging its tail.

I got up slowly. "Junior, I'm going to choke you."

He doubled over with squeals and chuckles. I wiped my filthy shorts with one hand and stretched out the other to snatch Junior's neck. The stupid little dog had the nerve to growl.

"Me and Thunder hid in the bushes. We followed you." He continued laughing. Then he turned to the dog. "Thunder, didn't Tasha look

---

3. mangy (MAYN gee) *adj.*: Dirty.

funny holding that stick like she was going to beat up the tree trunk?"

I put my hands around Junior's neck. "This is the end of the tail," I said.

Junior grinned. "You promised. 'I'll play any game he wants. I'll never yell at him again. I promise never to be mean to him again in my life.'"

Naomi giggled. "That's what you said, Tasha." The mutt barked at me. Guess he called himself Junior's protector. I took my hands off Junior's neck.

Then Naomi had a laughing spasm. She pointed at the dog. "Is that what everyone was running from?"

"This is my trusted guard. People say he's wild. He just wants a friend."

"Thunder looks like he's already got a lot of friends living inside his fur," I said. We walked back to the block with the dog trotting right by Junior's side.

I checked my watch when we got to my building. "It's ten to twelve. I have to make lunch for Junior," I told Naomi. "But I'll be back out later."

The dog whined after Junior as we entered the building. "I'll be back soon, Thunder," he said, "after I beat my sister in five games of checkers."

Now he was going to blackmail me.

I heard Naomi giggling as Junior and I walked into the building. The phone rang just as we entered the apartment. I knew it was Ma.

"Everything okay, Tasha? Nothing happened?"

"No, Ma, everything is fine. Nothing happened at all."

◆

Well, the summer didn't turn out to be so terrible after all. My parents got Thunder cleaned up and let Junior keep him for a pet. Me and my friends practiced for the double-dutch contest right in front of my building, so I didn't have to leave the block. After lunch when it was too hot to jump rope, I'd play a game of checkers with Junior or read him a story. He wasn't as pesty as he used to be, because now he had Thunder. We won the double-dutch contest. And Junior never told my parents that I'd lost him. I found out that you never miss a tail until you almost lose it.

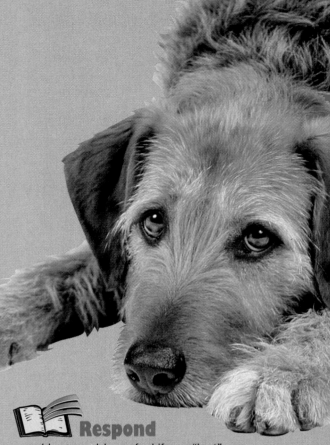

Respond

- How would you feel if you "lost" a young person you were baby-sitting? Explain.
- With classmates, role-play looking for the lost child. Include the thoughts you might have while the child was missing.

Joyce Hansen (1942–   ) knew she had to "find her own voice" in order to be the best writer she could be. "I sat down one day," she says, "and read over everything I had ever written. While doing this, it was as if everything I'd ever studied about writing made sense." It was then that Hansen began writing her first book.

Words to Know

spasm (SPAZ uhm) *n.:* A short, sudden burst
blackmail (BLAK mayl) *v.:* Threaten to tell something harmful about someone unless certain conditions are met

Explore Your Reading

Look Back (Recall)

1. List the ways that Tasha breaks her mother's rules.

Think It Over (Interpret)

2. Compare and contrast the ways that Naomi and Tasha act toward Junior. Include an explanation for the differences.
3. Why does Junior hide from Tasha?
4. What does Tasha mean when she says, "I found out that you never miss a tail until you almost lose one"? Explain.
5. How does Tasha's statement show a change in attitude?

Go Beyond (Apply)

6. Tasha learns some important things because of her experience. Explain which of them apply to your life as well.

Develop Reading and Literary Skills

Analyze Suspense

This story is filled with **suspense,** a nervous feeling that keeps you guessing, about the fate of Tasha's brother. As danger builds, you want to keep reading to find out how the problem is solved.

From the start, you know Tasha doesn't want to watch Junior. By the time they get to the park, you wonder if something terrible will happen. The story increases suspense by introducing frightening details. For example, the characters talk about a yellow dog with red eyes. By mentioning the yellow dog twice, the writer focuses your attention on a frightening image. The suspense increases as you imagine the dog hurting Junior.

1. Choose two of the incidents on your chart. Explain how they created suspense by raising questions in your mind.
2. Explain how the suspense in this story helps readers to understand the lesson that Tasha learns.

Ideas for Writing

Imagine that Tasha wants to remember and share what she has learned about the responsibilities of baby-sitting.

Baby-sitter's Journal As Tasha, write about the experiences that you had baby-sitting for Junior. Choose several days to describe and show how your attitude and behavior changed during the summer.

Editorial Take the role of Tasha and write an editorial for your school paper. Persuade your readers that young people should take care of their younger brothers and sisters. Use what you learned from babysitting for Junior to support your argument.

Ideas for Projects

Checklist In this story you learned some of the *dos* and *don't*s of babysitting. Create a baby-sitter's checklist that includes information that you need from parents, ideas for activities, and safety tips. Reproduce the checklist and give it to baby sitters and parents.

Illustrated Report Like Tasha, teenagers throughout history have had responsibilities that they must fulfill. Research the lives of teenagers during the Middle Ages. Find out about the tasks of pages and squires. Use social studies textbooks and reference books to help your research. Write up your findings and illustrate two or three of the responsibilities you think are interesting or unusual.

How Am I Doing?

Answer these questions to summarize what you've learned:

What have I learned about techniques of suspense that I can use to analyze television shows and movies?

How does this story help me understand how I decide what's right?

Activities PREVIEW

Sarah Cynthia Sylvia Stout Would Not Take the Garbage Out   by Shel Silverstein

Have you ever not wanted to do your chores?

Reach Into Your Background

You may have certain chores to do every day. You probably have to make your bed and put away your clothes. Perhaps you have to do the dishes after dinner or take out the garbage or walk the dog. If you're like most people, you probably don't enjoy all of your jobs, and you would rather not do them. Think about the chores that people your age do. Then do one or both of these activities with a small group:

- Make a chart of household tasks that most of your classmates do. Devise a system to rank your reactions to these chores. For example, you might give pleasant chores four stars.
- Tell a group story about someone who refused to do chores. Each person adds a sentence until the conflict is solved. Exaggerate—overstate—to add humor and emphasis to your story.

Read Actively

Identify Exaggeration

When people talk about something they really like or dislike, they often **exaggerate,** or overstate the truth, to make their point. Writers create humor by exaggerating ordinary situations and creating details that probably couldn't happen. Recognizing this technique can help you find the humor in a story or a poem.

As you read the poem, jot down the exaggerations that Shel Silverstein uses. Complete the chart to record your reactions to the exaggerations.

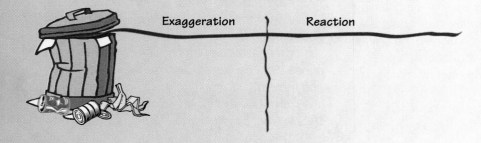

Exaggeration	Reaction

Sarah Cynthia Sylvia Stout Would Not Take the Garbage Out

Shel Silverstein

Sarah Cynthia Sylvia Stout
Would not take the garbage out!
She'd scour the pots and scrape the pans,
Candy the yams and spice the hams,
5   And though her daddy would scream and shout,
She simply would not take the garbage out.
And so it piled up to the ceilings:
Coffee grounds, potato peelings,
Brown bananas, rotten peas,
10 Chunks of sour cottage cheese.
It filled the can, it covered the floor,
It cracked the window and blocked the door
With bacon rinds and chicken bones,
Drippy ends of ice cream cones,
15 Prune pits, peach pits, orange peel,
Gloppy glumps of cold oatmeal,
Pizza crusts and withered greens,
Soggy beans and tangerines,
Crusts of black burned buttered toast,
20 Gristly bits of beefy roasts . . .
The garbage rolled on down the hall,
It raised the roof, it broke the wall . . .

Words to Know

scour (SKOWR) *v.*: Clean by rubbing vigorously (line 3)
candy (KAN dee) *v.*: Coat with sugar (line 4)
rinds (RĪNDZ) *n.*: Tough outer layers or skins (line 13)
withered (WITH uhrd) *adj.*: Dried up (line 17)

Greasy napkins, cookie crumbs,
Globs of gooey bubble gum,
25 Cellophane from green baloney,
Rubbery blubbery macaroni,
Peanut butter, caked and dry,
Curdled milk and crusts of pie,
Moldy melons, dried-up mustard,
30 Eggshells mixed with lemon custard,
Cold french fries and rancid meat,
Yellow lumps of Cream of Wheat.
At last the garbage reached so high
That finally it touched the sky.
35 And all the neighbors moved away,
And none of her friends would come to play.
And finally Sarah Cynthia Stout said,
"OK, I'll take the garbage out!"
But then, of course, it was too late . . .
40 The garbage reached across the state,
From New York to the Golden Gate
And there, in the garbage she did hate,
Poor Sarah met an awful fate,
That I cannot right now relate
45 Because the hour is much too late.
But children, remember Sarah Stout
And always take the garbage out!

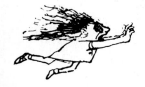

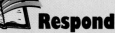

Respond

• What descriptions or images in this poem do you think are funny?
• With a partner, read the poem aloud slowly and then quickly. Discuss which reading style worked better.

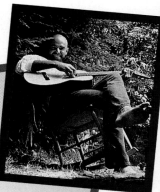

Shel Silverstein (1932–) is a poet, storyteller, songwriter, and artist.

THEN: "When I was a kid—I couldn't play ball, I couldn't dance. . . . The girls didn't want me . . . so I started to draw and write."

NOW: "I want to go everywhere, look at and listen to everything. You can go crazy with some of the wonderful stuff there is in life."

Activities

MAKE MEANING

Explore Your Reading

Look Back (Recall)

1. List five things that happen because Sarah Cynthia Sylvia Stout refused to take out the garbage.

Think It Over (Interpret)

2. When does the poem become unrealistic?
3. What do you think is the fate of Sarah Cynthia Sylvia Stout?
4. What is the purpose of the exaggeration in this poem?

Go Beyond (Apply)

5. How could you use this poem to help convince people to recycle?

Develop Reading and Literary Skills

Appreciate Humor in Poetry

By noticing exaggeration, you've already identified one basis for **humor,** the quality that makes something comical or amusing. Poets also use other techniques to help make readers laugh.

For example, Silverstein uses a cause-and-effect chain to show the outrageous results of Sarah's refusal to take out the garbage. In addition, he uses vivid words and fantastic details to create amusing images in your mind. Think about these humorous lines: "It filled the can, it covered the floor,/It cracked the window and blocked the door." The absurd picture they create adds to the humor.

The poet also uses rhyme, the repetition of like-sounding words at the ends of lines, to heighten the humor. "Green baloney" and "blubbery macaroni" may be disgusting, yet rhyme makes them funny.

1. List three vivid images that create humor.
2. Give an example of a rhyme that you find funny.
3. How do you know that Silverstein does not mean for you to take this poem seriously?

Ideas for Writing

This poem uses humor to point out an important idea. Choices have consequences and bad choices can have very negative consequences.

Feature Story For your school newspaper or a teen magazine, write a feature story that describes a day in the life of a teenager. Use a humorous style that shows the choices teenagers face each day and the consequences of those choices.

Poem Write a poem in the spirit of a tall tale or exaggerated story that tells what happened to someone who didn't do a chore. You may want to create a humorous sequel to this poem telling about the fate of Sarah Cynthia Sylvia Stout. Use your humor to help readers appreciate the meaning of your poem.

Ideas for Projects

Collage Use pictures from magazines, words from newspapers, and bits of other materials to create a collage that illustrates "Sarah Cynthia Sylvia Stout Would Not Take the Garbage Out."

A Statistical Report of the Environment One expert estimates that the average person in the United States discards three to four pounds of garbage each day. Check local resources to research more detailed statistics about refuse in your community. Use the average household as the base for your presentation. Then create a visual presentation such as a chart, graph, or picture story that shows the amount of garbage your community disposes of daily. [Math Link; Science Link]

How Am I Doing?

Take a moment to answer these questions in your journal:

How do I recognize humor?

What did this poem make me realize about the power of my own decisions?

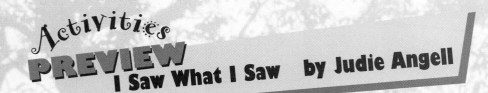

Activities
PREVIEW
I Saw What I Saw   by Judie Angell

Who is the wisest person you ever met?

Reach Into Your Background

Throughout your life, you've probably met many people who have taught you valuable lessons. Your teachers, your coaches, and your parents or grandparents are just a few sources of wisdom. The lady next door may have taught you to care for animals because she saved some stray cats. Through their words or actions, even strangers have a way of teaching others.

Consider the different people who teach you about life, and complete one or both of the following with a small group:

- Brainstorm for a list of the kinds of lessons you learn outside of school.
- Discuss the movies or television shows you've seen that show a younger person learning from a neighbor, friend, teacher, or stranger. Reenact important scenes that show the relationship.

Read Actively
Draw Conclusions About Characters

In real life, we learn about people through our interactions with them. We **draw conclusions** about others based on the things they say and do. You can use the same strategy when you read. Draw conclusions about **characters,** the people in stories, by using words and actions to tell you what the writer may not say about each character. If you draw conclusions about characters, you will get a fuller understanding of each one.

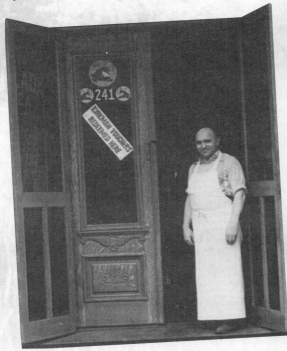

As you read, jot down notes about Ray Beane and Mr. Meyer, the two main characters in this story. Draw conclusions about each character and then consider what each gets out of a relationship with the other.

I Saw What I Saw

Judie Angell

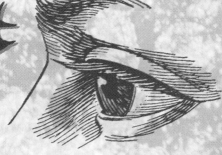

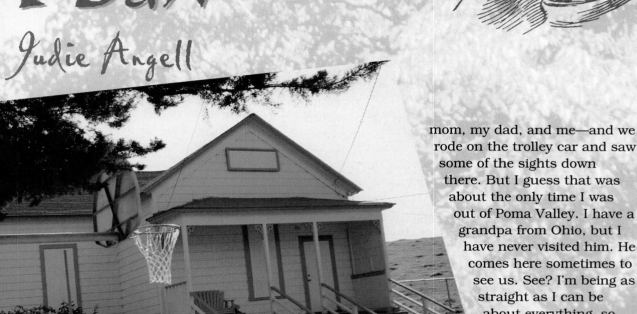

mom, my dad, and me—and we rode on the trolley car and saw some of the sights down there. But I guess that was about the only time I was out of Poma Valley. I have a grandpa from Ohio, but I have never visited him. He comes here sometimes to see us. See? I'm being as straight as I can be about everything, so nobody can say I lied or exaggerated or anything.

Yeah. Well. I'm not dumb. I don't lie, and I'm not one of those nuts, either. Ask anyone, anyone who's known me for the last twelve years, which is all the time I've been alive, if Ray Beane ever, I mean *ever* ran off at the mouth with stupid stuff nobody'd believe. I never did. I always tell it straight. My dad, before he died, that's the way he raised me. And my mom, she's the same way. *Be on the level with folks, Ray, and always look 'em in the eye.*

I live in Poma Valley, California. I was born here, like I said, twelve years ago, and I haven't hardly been anywhere else in all that time. Once, when I was nine—this was just before the Lord took my dad away with cancer—we went on a little trip south to San Francisco. It was just the three of us—my

Poma Valley is a little town. Very rural, you'd call it. Only about five thousand people. And I go to school in a one-room schoolhouse, just like that old-fashioned program you see sometimes in reruns on TV. It's true. We have

📖 **Read Actively**

Ask yourself what the writing style tells you about the narrator.

the sixth, seventh, and eighth grades all in one room. And there's only ten of us in all those classes. I get there by bus and it takes about forty-five minutes to an hour, depending on the roads and the weather. Cross my heart. I know there are a lot of people who won't believe there are really places like that left in America, but there are, and I live in one. It's real, all right.

I know what's real.

I told you my name, but the whole of it is

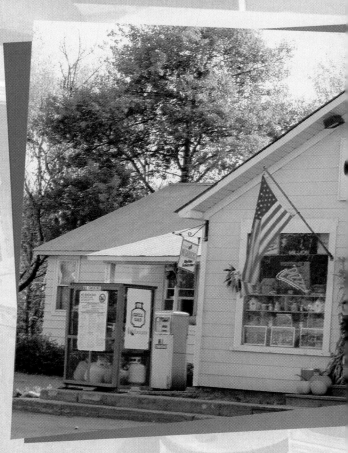

Raymond Earl Beane, Junior. I was named for my dad, and when I have a son of my own I'm going to name him Raymond Earle Beane the Third. My mom, she laughs and says I'd better have a wife who agrees with that choice, but I don't guess I'd marry somebody who didn't. Anyway, that's my name, and I said my age and mentioned everyone in my family except for some cousins who also live in Ohio, so that's it for my autobiography. We did autobiographies this year in seventh grade. Mine was pretty short.

I stand about five-two and weigh in at about one hundred ten. I'm not very big, but it doesn't bother me. I've got yellowish hair. It's straight and long, sort of, behind the ears. I like soccer and football and I like to listen to country music. Most of my friends like rock, but I like country, and I don't care who knows it.

I have a dog. Maybe I should have mentioned him as part of my family, but I'll mention him now. He's part Lab and his name's Red. He's a black dog, but his name's Red and that's it.

I guess that's enough about me, but I wanted to tell the kind of person I am to help prove out what I say. Hope nobody minds.

The time I'm talking about now, it was six months ago in May. Just getting on to summer. What I wanted real bad was a team jacket. For soccer. I was on the team, and all the other kids had red jackets that said "Poma Valley Soccer" in white on the back with a picture of a soccer ball, and then you got your first name in white script writing put on the front on the left side. Boy, I wanted one, but we just couldn't afford it, Mom and me. See, I had a good jacket, so I didn't really need another one. This was just something I wanted. Around our house we can really just about deal with what we need. "Want" is something else.

So Mom said if I could raise the money over the summer, it'd be okay with her if I bought myself that jacket. And what's when it started.

Our main street, well, it's called Main Street, and like you'd expect, it runs straight through town and then it turns into Route 34 and goes on to skirt by the farms. But there's a movie theater called The Poma on it, along with a pharmacy, a launderette, a Thom McAnn shoe store, a hardware store, and a few other shops I can't remember. Oh, right, there's an army-navy store, too, and a diner on the corner. Out a ways in the other direction, there's an A & P and a bowling alley, too, and that's about it for Poma Valley.

The store I didn't mention is the little market between the launderette and the pharmacy. It sells groceries. It's called Meyer's.

I started out looking for work in the bowling alley. I wasn't sure what I could do, but I thought it would be fun to hang out there and maybe get to bowl a few frames every now and then, you know, improve my game. But no luck. So I moved on to the shoe store and the pharmacy (I skipped the launderette—doing the laundry at home is bad enough). I didn't have any luck there either, and I finally ended up at Meyer's grocery store.

We never shopped at Meyer's. Mom says the little markets are always more expensive since they can't buy in bulk the way the supermarkets can, so I had never met Mr. Meyer before. I guess I'd seen him some. I mean, you can't really miss anyone who lives or works in Poma Valley, but I never paid him any mind before that day. Funny thing was, he knew me.

"Ray Beane," he says when I come in. And he grins this big grin at me. I guess my jaw kind of drops and he laughs. His laugh is big and nice, not the kind of laugh where you think maybe he's making fun of you. "Sure I know you," he says. "I like to know who all the kids are."

I found out later that it was true he liked most of the kids, but he also wanted to keep an eye on us. There are plenty of kids who take stuff, rip it off, you know. And if he knew kids, called them by name and treated them nice, maybe they wouldn't do it so much to him. Take stuff, I mean.

He was a smart man, Mr. Meyer, but I didn't find any of this stuff out till later. Till I started working for him and getting to know him.

Yeah, he hired me. Minimum wage[1] plus the tips I'd earn for deliveries. Part-time after school, and when school let out a few weeks later, full-time, ten till six. Sweep the place inside and out, dust the shelves, pack groceries, even wait on customers if he was busy, all the stuff you'd expect would be done in a small grocery store. What he didn't mention was he really wanted somebody to talk to. He talked a lot.

If that sounds as if I didn't like to hear him talk, then I said it wrong. I did like it.

Mr. Meyer's first name was Abe. Abraham. He was Jewish and spoke with an accent. He told me his age—sixty-seven.

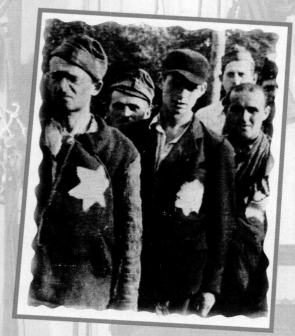

He was proud of it, he said, because he had been in a concentration camp[2] in the Second World War and any time he lived after that was "borrowed time." He laughed when he said it, but I knew he didn't think it was funny.

Except the thing is, he wasn't at all angry or anything, just grateful. He said he was grateful to have come out of such a dark and terrible time and be able to live in sunny California and run his own business, too.

He didn't have a family. He said they all died in the camp. He showed me two pictures, of a dark-haired woman and a little girl. The pictures were very old—they were black and white, and yellow around the edges, but he was proud of them and kept them in a gold frame in back of the counter.

"My mother," he said. "And my sister." He told me their names, but I couldn't pronounce them. I know that the only time his eyes didn't laugh was when he looked at those two pictures.

_____

1. **minimum wage:** The lowest rate of pay allowed by law.

_____

2. **concentration camp:** A prison camp where Nazis held Jews and others during World War II. Millions of Jews were brought to these camps and killed.

The truth was that the store wasn't that busy most of the time. A lot of people must be like my mom and they shop at the A & P. Some folks'd come in for last-minute things like a newspaper or a carton of milk or bread or something, but not too much more. I may have made—tops—three deliveries all summer. But lunchtime was busy. Mr. Meyer made deli sandwiches, and the guys who worked on the roads and the truckers and local folks would come in for tuna salad, bologna, roast beef, whatever, and milk or a soda or beer. I guess that's where most of the money was made, the lunches. Anyway, he never complained about money, Mr. Meyer, so I guess he made enough for his needs. I didn't complain either, because so did I. And then some.

Except for lunchtime, we had time to kill, Mr. Meyer and me. We'd sit down behind the counter and he'd give me what he called his "philosophy of life."

"There's always someone worse off than you, Ray Beane," he'd say. He always called me Ray Beane, my whole name, like it was one word. "It's sad you have no papa, but a mama you have. There are boys who don't have both, you know. And not only that, your mama, she loves you very much, right?"

"Well, yeah . . ."

"'Well, yeah,' you say. Of course she loves you very much. To have someone to love you is a wonderful thing."

I wanted to ask him who he had to love *him*, except I thought it would be rude. Only he was one step ahead of me there.

"When I was young, I had a whole big family who loved me very much, so I know what it's like. Many people, they never know what it is like to be loved."

I looked at him.

"It's like the optimist and the pessimist, yes? The optimist has a glass of water, he says it is half full. The pessimist has the same glass, he says it is half empty. You see the difference?"

I thought I did.

"When you wake up in the morning, Ray Beane, what do you see?" he asked.

I thought for a second.

"Uh . . . my alarm clock . . . my closet door . . . Red, lots of times, he wakes me up."

"Do you see the sunlight streaming through your window?"

"Uh, yeah . . ."

"'Uh, yeah.' Does it make you feel good that another day is here? Another day when you can put on your clothes and your shoes and walk around, healthy, in the sunlight?"

"Uh, yeah . . ."

"'Uh, yeah.' Some vocabulary you got there, Ray Beane. We got to do something about that."

"I got an A in Vocabulary," I told him.

He smiled. "Only old men think about being lucky to wake up in the sunshine and walk around," he said. "Kids don't have to think about that. But it would be nice if they did. Just once in a while, Ray Beane. Think about it. It will make you a nicer person."

I didn't see how, but I liked him, so I decided to think about it. Once in a while.

"Did you know, Ray Beane, that ninety-nine percent of the things you worry about never, never happen?" he asked once.

"Huh?"

"It's true. Ninety-nine percent. A fact."

"Sometimes they do," I said.

"One percent. The odds are very good that worrying is a waste of time. And besides, worrying won't change what happens anyway, will it?"

I shook my head.

He shrugged this big shrug. His shoulders covered his ears. "So why worry?"

That was the kind of stuff he said, all the time. I told Mom about him and the things he said, and she said he sounded like a very wise man. She still didn't shop there, though—she said everything in his place was at least a dime more than at the A & P.

Once my friend Frankie came in for candy. He was with his older brother and they were both acting wise. You know, kidding around, punching each other and ragging on us a little. Frankie was doing it because his brother Jim was there. Usually he's pretty nice. But anyway, I saw Jim lift this Baby Ruth bar off the candy rack. I caught him in the big round magnifying mirror Mr. Meyer has at the front of the store, so you can see what's going on in the aisles. I didn't know what to do. I mean it. If I said something, I'd be dead meat when school started—I knew it. But still, there was Mr. Meyer and how nice he was to me and all—I mean, I always got to take stuff home at the end of the day and he was teaching me things—he made me learn a fact from the encyclopedia every single day and memorize it and tell it to him. He did.

I couldn't stand it. I turned red and my stomach hurt and then before I even knew it, Frankie and Jim were gone, outta there. My stomach hurt worse than before, but I still didn't say anything. And then I felt a hand on my shoulder.

"It's okay, Ray Beane. I knew they were your friends."

I felt like I was about to cry. Okay, I did cry.

"You're my friend too," I blubbered, feeling like a total wuss.

"A different kind," he said.

"Well, if you saw, how come you didn't say anything?" I asked, wiping my nose on my sleeve and feeling even stupider.

He didn't answer. I knew it was because he was waiting to see what I would do.

"I won't let it go again," I said, real softly.

"I won't put you in that position again," he said, even softer.

Later, after work, I found Frankie. I told him if he ever came in there with Jim again and ripped off Mr. Meyer, I'd personally break his face. I said *his,* not Jim's, because I couldn't take Jim. But I can take Frankie and he knows it, so it was a personal thing, between the two of us, and that way no one at school would have to know and Mr. Meyer wouldn't have to know and Frankie wouldn't let it happen again. I guessed. I hoped. I sort of worried about it every time Frankie came into the store with his brother, which wasn't even that often, but neither of them even flicked a whisker, so Mr. Meyer was right about that—I worried for nothing.

It was what I *didn't* worry about that happened.

It was a Thursday. I know it was a Thursday. I woke up and thought about the sunshine that day. I was grinning all the way to work and I told Mr. Meyer about it, and he grinned too. And the day was bright and nice like it usually is, especially in summer. It was morning, before the lunch folks, so the store had its usual few customers. I remember Mrs. Lefton came in and bought cat food and Mrs. Crowley came in for orange juice and bread—she's the housekeeper for old Mr. Staley—and Willy Pelosi bought a paper, two doughnuts, and a black coffee. I remember all of that.

And I remember the truck. It was a red pickup and it pulled up right in front of

> 📖 **Read Actively**
> **Predict** what kind of event will happen.

the store, right there in the sunshine on Main Street, and one man jumped out of it. He was wearing a hat. And then it was fast and blurry and I don't like to talk about it, but this is the way it went.

The man had a gun and he pointed it right at us, Mr. Meyer and me. And he said he wanted money. He knew the old man kept a lot of it in a vault[3] in the back and he wanted it, he wanted it. Mr. Meyer never said a word, but he was holding a can of bug spray—we were stacking them, the ant-and-roach-killer cans; he said they do pretty well in summer— and he suddenly threw it, the can, he *threw* it right at the guy with the gun. He hit the guy and the guy dropped the gun, but not before it went off. And then Mr. Meyer, he picked up another spray can and sprayed the guy's face. The guy was yelling, because of the spray in his face, and I was so scared, I mean, I hope and pray never to be so scared again, but there was Mr. Meyer right next to me, saying, "It's okay, Ray Beane, get the gun, now before he can see again, that's the boy, that's my boy, now hold it on him, I'm right here, we'll hold it on him, we'll do it together, just like we do things."

And he winked at me. He really did. Winked at me. I saw it.

Then I was holding the gun and hollering my head off. Outside I could hear the truck pulling away, grinding gears and blowing soot, and then Mr. Aiken from the pharmacy came in and he was with a whole bunch of people who heard the gun and the yelling and the truck and everything, and the police came and they took the guy away. He was still covering his face and crying or something from the spray in his eyes.

---

3. vault (VAWLT) *n.*: A large safe for keeping valuables.

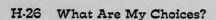

And then Mr. Aiken, he put his arm around my shoulders and took me out of the store. Darned if I wasn't crying again, but I was shaking so bad I could hardly stand, I was still so scared.

"It's okay, Raymond. They've called your mom and she's on her way. It's all right, boy, it's all right," he kept saying.

And the crowd, I could hear the crowd. It was too early for the lunch folks, but they were there anyway—they just appeared, along with the rest of Poma Valley. I remember it all just perfectly, just like it was going on right this minute.

"Nothing like this *ever* happened before in the valley . . ."

"Did too. Last year and the year before."

"That was the gas station got held up. And it was at night, no one was there."

"Was too there."

"Was not and there weren't no gun."

"One of 'em got away."

"Yeah, in a red pickup. They'll get him."

"Poor kid, poor Ray."

"Ray's the lucky one. Poor Meyer, that's who. Poor old guy."

That's when I stopped blubbering.

"What about Mr. Meyer?" I asked.

But instead of answering me, Mr. Aiken just kept patting and squeezing my shoulder. I moved quickly, then, and started to head back into the store, but Mr. Aiken and someone else grabbed me and held on to me and wouldn't let me go. So I *really* started hollering then, you bet, just yelling my fool head off for Mr. Meyer to come out. *"Come out! Mr. Meyer! Come out! Come out, Mr. Meyer!"*

But "Shh, boy" was all Mr. Aiken would say, and everyone else just seemed to turn away from us, looking down at the sidewalk or up the street into the sun.

"He can't come out, Ray," Mrs. Lefton said. She took Mr. Aiken's place and pulled me away with her arm around my shoulder. "He can't come out, Ray, honey, he was shot. That shot everyone heard, it caught him, honey. You don't want to go back in there—"

But I did, and she couldn't hold me then. Nobody could. I raced past them, pushed past them. There wasn't anybody who could stop me then.

The paramedics from the volunteer ambulance corps were picking him up from where he'd been lying on the floor at the end of the shelf with all the bug sprays. They put him on a gurney,[4] and even though I knew he was dead, I still lost it when I saw them put the sheet over him.

They did catch the guy in the truck. His pal told them just where to find him. He also said how he heard "the old guy" had this safe in back of his store with all this money, and how he knew the store was never busy that time of day, all kinds of stupid and weird stuff like that. I'm trying to say how I remember it all, and I do, anyone can see that, but it didn't come together for me until the police questioned me later. Actually, it was just Captain Ebsen, who sometimes takes my mother out, both of them being widowed. It was when he was asking me all those questions that everyone started looking at me funny.

See, the gun went off just once, and that's when Mr. Meyer had to have been shot. But it

---

4. **gurney** (GER nee) *n.*: A stretcher on wheels.

Words to Know

rational (RASH uh nuhl) *adj.*: Logical; able to reason

was *after* the gun went off that he sprayed the robber's face and told me to hold the gun on him and said we'd do it together, that he was with me. And winked at me.

But everyone said I was too upset to be rational. That's what they said. I wasn't rational, but it was understandable, they said, after what I went through.

Well, yeah, I guess I went through something. And I guess he'll always be with me, that old man and his old pictures and his "philosophy of life." And I don't guess I'll ever really get over what happened to him. I'll remember everything he said about being lucky and about worrying and about the sunshine and about the half-full glass, just like I know he'd want me to.

But after that shot went off, he was *there* next to me, calling me Ray Beane and telling me we'd do it together.

And he winked at me.

I saw what I saw.

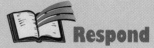 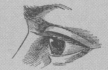

Respond

- Imagine you are Ray Beane. What are your feelings as the story ends?
- Choose a moment in the story in which Ray has to make a decision. Consider the end, or the time he sees his friends stealing. With a partner, discuss the decisions you might have made.

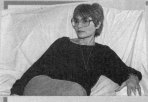

Judie Angell (1937–) "I think growing up heads the list of The Hardest Things To Do In Life. It's so hard in fact, that some of us never get there. But even with the world changing as rapidly as it does, the feelings that we have while we're coping with those changes don't," says Judie Angell. Angell was born in New York City and taught elementary school before she started writing stories for young adults.

MAKE MEANING

Explore Your Reading

Look Back (Recall)

1. List three important facts about Ray Beane's life before he met Mr. Meyer.

Think It Over (Interpret)

2. Why do you think Ray likes Mr. Meyer?
3. Explain how you know that Mr. Meyer is an optimist.
4. Why is the relationship between Ray and Mr. Meyer good for both of them?
5. How do you explain what happens at the end of the story?

Go Beyond (Apply)

6. How could a friend like Mr. Meyer help you with some of your life's choices?

Develop Reading and Literary Skills

Understand the Theme Through Character

Your notes about Ray and Mr. Meyer probably show that they had a very good relationship even though they were from very different backgrounds. How they act with each other gives you clues about who they are. **Characters,** the people in a story, and their relationships are often the key to the **theme,** a story's central message.

Like many stories, "I Saw What I Saw" has an implied theme. Angell does not tell you the message; you must figure it out. Use what you know about the relationship of Ray Beane and Mr. Meyer to analyze the story's theme. For example, Ray had lost his father and Mr. Meyer had lost his family, so they fill a gap in each other's lives. Ray liked Mr. Meyer because he treated Ray not as a child but as a human being. By analyzing Ray and Mr. Meyer and their relationship this way, you will discover the meaning of the story.

1. List three events from the story to show that Ray and Mr. Meyer had a positive relationship.
2. In what ways does Ray change after he meets Mr. Meyer?
3. What can readers learn from this story?

Ideas for Writing

Despite their very different backgrounds, Ray Beane and Mr. Meyer teach each other valuable lessons.

Anecdote Write a brief story about a person who has taught you or someone close to you a great deal. Focus on an interesting, amusing, or strange event in which you or the person you know learned an important lesson. Wherever possible, create dialogue to help tell the story.

Eulogy As Ray, write a speech that you will give at Mr. Meyer's funeral. In the speech give listeners enough detail to understand the relationship that you and Mr. Meyer had.

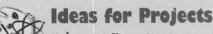

Ideas for Projects

Holocaust Report What could you learn from a Holocaust survivor? If you can meet with a survivor through a local synagogue or a Jewish organization such as B'nai B'rith, prepare questions that ask about the person's experiences and philosophy today. If no one is available to interview, use the library or the Internet to research biographies of Holocaust survivors. Write your findings in the form of a magazine question-and-answer article. [Social Studies Link]

Science Report Find out how a scientist would explain what Ray Beane says he saw. At the end of this story, Ray Beane insists he saw, talked to, and took instructions from Mr. Meyer even though the older man had been fatally shot. Begin by researching human senses and perception. Share your research with your classmates. [Science Link]

How Am I Doing?

Discuss these questions with a partner:

What did I learn about characters that helped me understand the story better? How can I apply what I learned to other kinds of literature?

Which example of my work will I put in my portfolio? What does it show I learned?

How can you put your dreams to the test?

Reach Into Your Background

Like most people, you probably have ideas and dreams for your future. You must make choices now to reach your goals later. There may be sacrifices to make. There may be hard work to do. However, if your hard work pays off, success will be yours. Think about your goals. Then explore your dreams by doing one or both of the following:

- In a group, discuss your dreams and aspirations. Talk about what each of you must do to achieve your goals.
- With a partner, role-play the first step you might take to put your dream in action. Think of what that step might be. Consider a telephone call, an interview, or a tryout.

Read Actively

Connect an Essay to Your Experience

When you **connect** what you read to your experience, you look for details and events in a selection that are in some way similar to those in your life. As you read **essays,** or short works of nonfiction, you might pause over a passage and wonder, "Would I do the same thing?" or "Do I know someone like that?" Connecting an essay to your experience will help you relate better to the writer's experiences and help you learn lessons that you can apply to your life.

In this essay, Alex Haley explains how he held on to his dreams even though it was difficult. As you read, fill in a chart like the one below. In the first column, record the events that led Haley to success. In the second column, tell what you might have done in a similar situation.

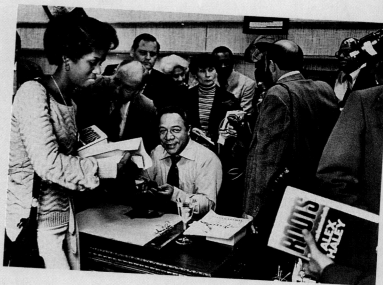

In 1976, the writer signs copies of his Pulitzer Prize winning book, *Roots.*

Alex Haley's Experience	What I Might Have Done

THE SHADOWLAND OF DREAMS

A l e x   H a l e y

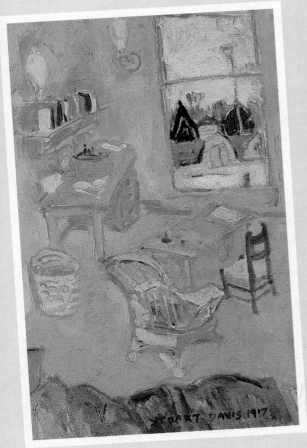

Studio Interior, 1917 (detail) Stuart Davis, Metropolitan Museum of Art/©1996 Estate of Stuart Davis/Licensed by VAGA, New York, New York

Many a young person tells me he wants to be a writer. I always encourage such people, but I also explain that there's a big difference between "being a writer" and writing. In most cases these individuals are dreaming of wealth and fame, not the long hours alone at a typewriter. "You've

Words to Know

neglect (ni GLEKT) *n*.: A lack of attention

got to want to *write*," I say to them, "not want to be a *writer*."

The reality is that writing is a lonely, private and poor-paying affair. For every writer kissed by fortune there are thousands more whose longing is never requited.[1] Even those who succeed often know long periods of neglect and poverty. I did.

When I left a 20-year-career in the Coast Guard to become a freelance writer,[2] I had no prospects at all. What I did have was a friend in New York City, George Sims, with whom I'd grown up in Henning, Tenn. George found me my home, a cleaned-out storage room in the Greenwich Village apartment building where he worked as superintendent. It didn't even matter that it was cold and had no bathroom. I immediately bought a used manual typewriter and felt like a genuine writer.

After a year or so, however, I still hadn't gotten a break and began to doubt myself. It was so hard to sell a story that I barely made enough to eat. But I knew I wanted to write. I had dreamed about it for years. I wasn't going to be one of those people who die wondering, *What if?* I would keep putting my dream to the test—even though it meant living with uncertainty and fear of failure. This is the Shadowland of hope, and anyone with a dream must learn to live there.

Then one day I got a call that changed my life. It wasn't an agent or editor offering a big contract. It was the opposite—a kind of siren call tempting me to give up my dream. On the phone was an old acquaintance from the Coast Guard, now stationed in San

---

1. requited (ree KWIT id) *v*.: Returned; rewarded.
2. freelance (FREE lans) **writer** *n*.: A writer who sells work to different buyers at different times.

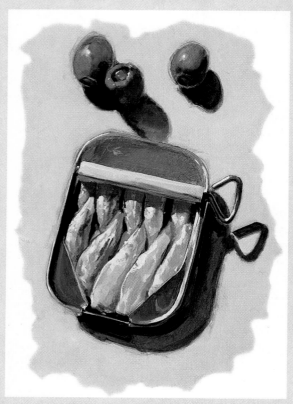

Sardines and Olives Francis Livingston, Jerry Leff Associates, Inc.

Francisco. He had once lent me a few bucks and liked to egg me about it. "When am I going to get that $15, Alex?" he teased.

"Next time I make a sale."

"I have a better idea," he said. "We need a new public-information assistant out here, and we're paying $6000 a year. If you want it, you can have it."

Six thousand a year! That was real money in 1960. I could get a nice apartment, a used car, pay off debts and maybe save a little something. What's more, I could write on the side.

As the dollars were dancing in my head, something cleared my senses. From deep inside a bull-headed resolution welled up. I

Words to Know

veteran (VET uhr uhn) *adj.*: Experienced
exhilarating (eg ZIL uh rayt ing) *adj.*: Exciting; lively

had dreamed of being a writer—full time. And that's what I was going to be. "Thanks, but no," I heard myself saying. "I'm going to stick it out and write."

Afterward, as I paced around my little room, I started to feel like a fool. Reaching into my cupboard—an orange crate nailed to the wall—I pulled out all that was there: two cans of sardines. Plunging my hands into my pockets, I came up with 18 cents. I took the cans and coins and jammed them into a crumpled paper bag. *There, Alex,* I said to myself. *There's everything you've made of yourself so far.* I'm not sure I've ever felt so low.

I wish I could say things started getting better right away. But they didn't. Thank goodness I had George to help me over the rough spots.

Through him I met other struggling artists like Joe Delaney, a veteran painter from Knoxville, Tenn. Often Joe lacked food money, so he'd visit a neighborhood butcher who would give him big bones with morsels of meat and a grocer who would hand him some wilted vegetables. That's all Joe needed to make down-home soup.

Another Village neighbor was a handsome young singer who ran a struggling restaurant. Rumor had it that if a customer ordered steak the singer would dash to a supermarket across the street to buy one. His name was Harry Belafonte.[3]

People like Delaney and Belafonte became role models for me. I learned that you had to make sacrifices and live creatively to keep working at your dream. That's what living in the Shadowland is all about.

As I absorbed the lesson, I gradually began to sell my articles. I was writing about what many people were talking about then: civil rights, black Americans and Africa. Soon, like birds flying south, my thoughts were drawn back to my childhood. In the silence of my room, I heard the voices of

---

3. **Harry Belafonte** (bel uh FAHN tee) (1927–): American singer and actor who became a popular folk-music star in the 1950's. He has also appeared in films.

Grandma, Cousin Georgia, Aunt Plus, Aunt Liz and Aunt Till as they told stories about our family and slavery.

These were stories that black Americans had tended to avoid before, and so I mostly kept them to myself. But one day at lunch with editors of Reader's Digest I told these stories of my grandmother and aunts and cousins; and I said that I had a dream to trace my family's history to the first African brought to these shores in chains. I left that lunch with a contract that would help support my research and writing for nine years.

It was a long, slow climb out of the shadows. Yet in 1976, 17 years after I left the Coast Guard, *Roots* was published. Instantly I had the kind of fame and success that few writers ever experience. The shadows had turned into dazzling limelight.

For the first time I had money and open doors everywhere. The phone rang all the time with new friends and new deals. I packed up and moved to Los Angeles, where I could help in the making of the *Roots* TV mini-series. It was a confusing, exhilarating time, and in a sense I was blinded by the light of my success.

Then one day, while unpacking, I came across a box filled with things I had owned years before in the Village. Inside was a brown paper bag.

I opened it, and there were two corroded[4] sardine cans, a nickel, a dime and three pennies. Suddenly the past came flooding in like a riptide. I could picture myself once again huddled over the typewriter in that cold, bleak, one-room apartment. And I said to myself, *The things in this bag are part of my roots too. I can't ever forget that.*

I sent them out to be framed in Lucite. I keep that clear plastic case where I can see it every day. I can see it now above my office desk in Knoxville, along with the Pulitzer Prize; a portrait of nine Emmys awarded the TV production of *Roots*; and the Spingarn medal—the NAACP's highest honor. I'd be hard pressed to say which means the most to me. But only one reminds me of the courage and persistence it takes to stay the course in the Shadowland.

It's a lesson anyone with a dream should learn.

———————
4. **corroded** (kuh ROH did): Rusted; worn away.

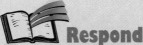

Respond

- What surprised you most about Alex Haley's experiences as a beginning writer?
- With a partner, list the items that you would put in a Lucite frame to help you remember your goals.

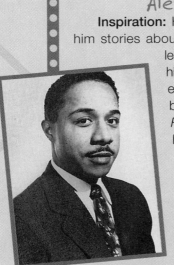

Alex Haley (1921–1992)

Inspiration: Haley's grandmother used to tell him stories about his ancestors. He decided to learn about his heritage and traced his family's history back seven generations to Africa. Haley later based his most famous book, *Roots*, and some others on what he learned in his research.

Favorite Writing Topics: He once said that while his most famous writing was about *his* family, writing about families is like writing about "every person on earth—we all have a family."

Explore Your Reading
Look Back (Recall)

1. What steps does Alex Haley take to pursue his dream?

Think It Over (Interpret)

2. What is the conflict that Haley faced?
3. Explain why he made the choice he did.
4. Why does Haley title this essay "The Shadowland of Dreams"?
5. Evaluate the decision Haley made. Consider the risks he took and the other options he had and then explain whether you think he made the right choice.

Go Beyond (Apply)

6. What advice do you think Haley would give young people about achieving their goals?

Develop Reading and Literary Skills
Respond to a Personal Essay

When you read a **personal essay**, a short account of a writer's true experiences, your own experiences and reactions help you relate to the author's message. Personal essays usually include the following elements:

- an informal, conversational style
- the writer's thoughts about one subject
- a message for readers to think about

Haley uses these elements to let readers know about a specific and private part of his life. By bringing readers into his decision-making process, Haley shares his struggles as a young writer. As you read, you may have wondered what choices he would make.

Use details from your chart to help you complete these activities:

1. Identify two vivid experiences Haley includes. Explain how each is important to the subject of the essay.

2. Find an example of the informal style Haley uses to communciate with readers.
3. What are the lessons Haley wants to share?

Ideas for Writing

Alex Haley dreamed of becoming a writer. What are some of your own goals and dreams?

Personal Essay In your own personal essay, discuss how you will fulfill an important dream. Use an informal style and a friendly approach. Include details about your personal experiences to make your message clear.

Short Story Create a story that shows a character trying to achieve a goal. If you like, base your story on Haley's experience. Since a story is fiction, you can change the facts, create details, and invent characters to make the story come alive.

Ideas for Projects

Goals Book As a class, create a book that records each class member's dreams and aspirations. Include photographs or drawings, a quotation that expresses something important about each student, and a paragraph or two describing the dreams and goals of your classmates. Keep the dream book in your class as a resource.

Song With others or by yourself, write a song about fulfilling your dreams. You can create an original tune or use a melody that already exists. Record your song or perform it for the class. [Music Link]

How Am I Doing?

Take a moment to respond to these questions:
What did I learn from Alex Haley's personal essay? How can I apply it to my life?
What informal goals do I want to set for myself?

What Are My Choices?

Think Critically About the Selections

All of the selections in this section focus on the question "What are my choices?" With a partner or a small group, complete one or two of the following activities to show what you've learned. You can write your responses in a journal or share them in discussion.

1. Imagine that two characters from the section were talking with you about the decisions that they made. Create a dialogue in which two characters from different selections discuss the reasons for their choices and how those choices changed their lives. Include advice they might give you about your decisions. **(Summarize; Hypothesize)**

2. Graduation speakers are chosen because they can inspire the audience. Select one of the characters from this section to be a speaker at your graduation. What inspiring message would this character give your classmates? **(Evaluate; Draw Conclusions)**

3. Which selection taught you something about deciding what choices are right? What did you learn from the selection? **(Synthesize)**

4. Look at the art on this page. How do you think the artist would answer the question "What are my choices?" Why? **(Make Inferences; Provide Evidence)**

Projects

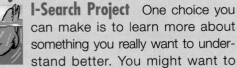

I-Search Project One choice you can make is to learn more about something you really want to understand better. You might want to study sign language, dolphins, or the stock exchange. Once you have your topic, find experts and collect materials. Read newspapers, books, and magazines. Give a presen-

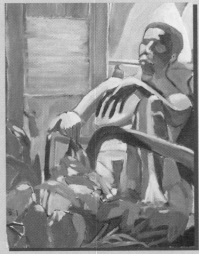

Student Art *Untitled* Guevera Soliman, Walt Whitman High School, Bethesda, Maryland

tation that tells the story of your research. Tell classmates how you became interested, what steps you took to pursue your interest, and what you learned.

Personal Interview With Career Professionals Conduct interviews with people who have jobs that interest you. Talk to people who work in areas related to math, science, social studies, and the arts. Prepare questions to discover how each made his or her career choice. Present the results of the interviews to the class. [Social Studies Link; Math Link; Science Link]

Multimedia Presentation: Choices Collect pictures, words, and music that relate to choices people your age have to make. Include the daily decisions you face as well as the larger choices you make. If possible, include videotaped sequences, slides, and recordings.

Looking at Folk

Rudolfo Anaya

Terms to know

A **folk tale** is an ancient story passed from one generation to the next by word of mouth. Many folk tales contain animals that talk, but folk tales can also feature ordinary humans. One of the best-loved characters in folk tales is the **trickster**, who relies on brains rather than strength or speed for success.

Deciding What's Right We have all been in situations when we had to decide what's right. How do we learn how to make difficult choices? Perhaps there are some common sense lessons in the folk tales we read.

King Solomon Wise King Solomon had to decide a very difficult case. There were two women, and each claimed to be the mother of the same child. They took their case to King Solomon.

King Solomon pondered the problem. Finally he said he would cut the child in two and give each woman half a child. The *real* mother of the child couldn't bear to see her child killed, so she told the king to give the child to the other woman. In this way King Solomon knew who the real mother was.

You may not be called on to solve a conflict this serious, but each day you have to make important choices about getting along with others and knowing what's right for you. Believe it or not, folk tales may help you decide.

How Do We Know What's Right? All groups of people make rules to live by. In "The Judgment of the Wind" the natural world gets involved in making an important decision. A man asks the wind, a tree, and other natural elements to help him resolve a conflict. In "Children of Wax," an ambitious boy takes his chances when he breaks a rule he has obeyed all his life.

In order to live in a civilized society we make laws that help us resolve conflicts. The men who wrote the Constitution of the United States used common sense. They had gained a lot of wisdom from the stories of their ancestors. Human nature and common sense help us make rules.

Even school has its set of rules. When we break a rule, we create conflict, then we have to resolve the problem. Usually we have to decide what's right on our own.

So How Does One Decide? Family and school help one decide what's right. So do good friends. Another way is to read stories in which the characters have to make the right choice. Folk tales make you think, and they help you apply common sense to your personal conflicts.

There are many folk tales in which the main character has to decide what's right.

Literary Forms
Tales

When you read these stories, think about how other characters influence the decision. Notice if anyone is hurt by the decision. Keep your attention focused by checking if the main character learns a lesson.

When the conflict is solved at the end of the story, we call that a resolution. When you read folk tales, you can compare some of the resolutions in the folk tales with resolutions you would have made. Your reactions may help you see your own ideas about what is right.

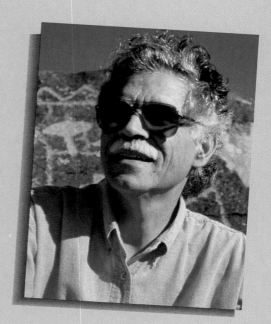

When **Rudolfo Anaya** (1937–   ) was young, he fell into an irrigation ditch near his Albuquerque home. He spent a long time in the hospital recovering from his spinal injury and returned home with a cane. During his recuperation, he spent many hours alone. Later, his writing allowed him a chance to express some of his loneliness. Anaya used his hospital experiences as the basis for his novel *Tortuga.*

In addition to his own writing, Anaya has published collections of folk tales of Mexico and the Southwest.

The Judgment of the Wind
by Harold Courlander and Wolf Leslau

How do we decide who's right and who's wrong?

Reach Into Your Background

Whether it's a courtroom rerun on TV or the most popular movie of the year, we seem to love a story about an exciting trial. People from earlier times also enjoyed stories that examined conflicting versions of what is right. For example, the question of what is right and wrong is a common subject of folk tales, stories passed from generation to generation by word of mouth.

Explore your ideas about what is right by doing one or more of these activities:

- In your journal, identify elements of nature that might be on opposite sides at a trial. For example, you might imagine what the coastline would say about a storm. Explain what each side would say.
- With a group, use what you know from TV and the movies to demonstrate what happens in trials. Role-play the people involved and act out the steps in the process.

Read Actively
Gather Evidence About a Conflict

You can't have a trial without opponents. This folk tale deals with opposing forces, too—a human being versus creatures in nature. Folk tales often explore what is right by presenting a **conflict,** or a struggle between opposing forces or characters. As you uncover the details of the conflict, you learn important clues about the plot, the characters, and the point of a folk tale.

Be a detective and investigate the facts as you read this folk tale. Gather evidence about the conflict and note it in your journal. Include whether you agree with the conclusions of the characters.

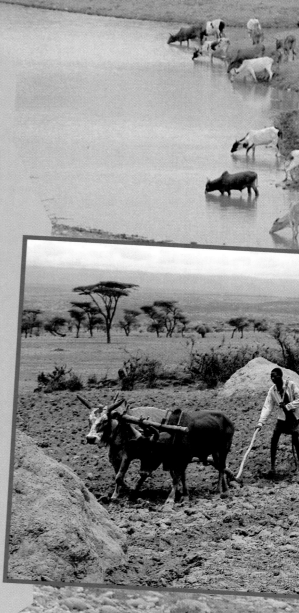

The Judgment of the Wind

Harold Courlander and Wolf Leslau

A great snake hid in the forest and preyed upon many living creatures who happened to pass his way. He sometimes went out of the forest and ate goats and cattle of villagers who lived nearby. At last a party of hunters went out to destroy him so that their cattle would be safe. With their spears and shields and hunting knives in their hands they looked for the snake where they found signs of him. Hearing them approach, he fled into a cotton field where a farmer was working.

The farmer was about to drop his tools and run away, but the snake said: "Brother, enemies are following me to kill me. Hide me so that I shan't die."

The farmer thought for a moment and then said:

"Though you have a bad reputation, one must have sympathy for the hunted."

And he hid the snake in a large pile of cotton standing in his field. When the hunters came along they asked:

"Have you seen the serpent that kills our cattle?"

"I have not seen him," the farmer replied, and the hunters went on.

The snake came out from under the cotton.

"They are gone," the farmer said. "You are safe."

But the snake did not go away. He took hold of the farmer.

"What are you doing?" the farmer asked.

"I am hungry," the snake said. "I shall have to eat you."

"What? I save your life and then you wish to destroy mine?"

"I am hungry," the snake replied. "I have no choice."

"You are ungrateful," the farmer said.

"I am hungry," the snake said.

"Since it is like this, let us have our case judged," the farmer said.

"Very well. Let the tree judge us."

So they went before the huge sycamore tree which grew at the side of the road. Each of them stated his case, while the tree listened.

Then the tree said to the farmer:

"I stand here at the edge of the road and give shade. Tired travelers come and sit in my shade to rest. And then when they are through they cut off my branches to make ax handles and plows. Man is ungrateful for the good I do him. Therefore, since it is

📖 Read Actively

Ask yourself who you think is right.

Words to Know

preyed (PRAYD) *v.*: Hunted other animals for food
reputation (rep yoo TAY shun) *n.*: What people generally think about the character of someone else

this way, I cannot judge in your favor. The snake is entitled to eat you."

The snake and the man went then to the river, and again they told their story. The river listened, and then it said to the farmer:

"I flow here between my banks and provide man with water. Without me, man would suffer; he would not have enough to drink. In the dry season when there are no rains, man comes and digs holes in my bed to find water for himself and his cattle. But when the heavy rains come I am filled to the brink. I cannot hold so much water, and I overflow onto man's fields. Then man becomes angry. He comes to me and curses me and throws stones at me. He forgets the good I do him. I have no use for man. Therefore, since this is man's nature, I cannot judge in your favor. The snake may eat you."

The snake and the man went to the grass, and once more they told their story. The grass listened, and then it said to the farmer:

"I grow here in the valley and provide food for man's cattle. I give myself to man to make roofs for his houses, and to make baskets for his kitchen. But then man puts the torch to me when I am old, and burns me. And after that he plows me under and plants grain in my place, and wherever I grow among the grain he digs me out and kills me. Man is not good. Therefore, I cannot judge in your favor. The snake may eat you."

The snake took hold of the farmer and they went away from the grass.

"The judgment is very cruel," the farmer said.

But on the road they met the wind. And though he had no hope, the farmer once more told his story. The wind listened, and then it said:

"All things live according to their nature. The grass grows to live and man burns it to live. The river flows to live, and overflows its banks because that is its nature; it cannot help it. And man grieves[1] when his planted fields are flooded, for they are his life. The tree cherishes its branches because they are its beauty. And the snake eats whatever it finds, for that, too, is his nature. So you see

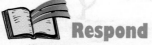

Read Actively

Gather evidence about the conflict. What facts can you find here?

one cannot blame the tree, the grass, and the river for their judgment, nor can one blame the snake for his hunger."

The farmer became even more sad, for he saw no way out for him. But the wind went on:

"So this is not a matter for judgment at all, but for all things acting according to their nature. Therefore, let us dance and sing in thanks because all things are as they are."

And the wind gave the farmer a drum to play, and he gave the snake a drum to play also. In order to hold his drum the snake had to let go of the farmer.

"As your nature is to eat man, eat man," the wind sang to the snake.

The wind turned to the farmer:

"As your nature is not to be eaten, do not be eaten!" it sang.

"Amen!" the farmer replied with feeling. And as the snake was no longer holding him, he threw down his drum and fled safely to his village.

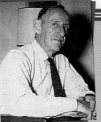

Respond

- If you were the farmer, how would you feel during your trials?
- Discuss with a group which character's judgment seemed the most fair and reasonable and why.

Harold Courlander's (1908–) father was a primitive painter. That helped to interest Courlander in the art of other cultures. Through his writing, he has worked especially hard to bring the legends and folk tales of different peoples to the rest of the world.

Wolf Leslau (LES law) has studied languages that were unknown to the rest of the world. Once, after months of research in Africa, he discovered a group of four people who were the last in the world who still spoke their language. His research has helped to preserve the history that can be found in the languages of many cultures.

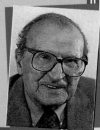

---

1. **grieves** (GREEVZ) *v.*: Feels deep sadness or grief.

Activities
MAKE MEANING

Explore Your Reading
Look Back (Recall)

1. What is the decision of most of the judges?

Think It Over (Interpret)

2. What opinion of human beings do most of the judges have? Explain.
3. Explain how the wind's judgment is different from the others.
4. In what ways are the judgments correct and in what ways are they unfair?

Go Beyond (Apply)

5. Compare and contrast the trial in this folk tale with trials in real courts of law.

Develop Reading and Literary Skills
Analyze Conflict in a Folk Tale

Your detective's notes probably show that there was a clash between the farmer and most of the other characters. This struggle between opposing forces or characters is the **conflict.** It is one of the most important elements of a story because it is the engine that drives the events of the plot.

The conflict in this **folk tale** from Eritrea and Ethiopia involves a human being fighting with nature. Each trial provides another reason to deny the farmer's request. For example, the tree points out that people are not thankful for all the good things they get from it. Therefore, the farmer deserves an unfavorable decision. Readers wonder if the farmer can possibly win. When the conflict is resolved, you learn the message of the folk tale.

1. Choose two judgments in the story and explain how each adds to the conflict.
2. What message does the resolution convey?
3. How does understanding the conflict in this folk tale help you to recognize its message?

Ideas for Writing

Folk tales often present conflicting ideas as legal disputes between rival creatures or elements. You can learn about ideas of right, wrong, and truth by examining each case.

Legal Brief Lawyers write legal briefs, or short statements that outline major arguments and evidence, and give them to the judge to consider. Develop a legal brief that outlines the major points of one of the characters in "The Judgment of the Wind."

Folk Tale Write your own folk tale that presents a truth by examining opposing arguments of rival creatures or elements. For example, you might show the conflict between the ocean and the shore or an argument between the wind and the rain.

Ideas for Projects

Folk-Tale Anthology With a group, create a collection of folk tales in which conflicting claims are settled. Include stories from different parts of the world and create illustrations for each one. [Social Studies Link]

Dance Create a dance that tells the story of this folk tale. Have the dancers move like each of the characters in the story. For example, the snake might slither and the tree might sway. Perform the dance for the class.

How Am I Doing?

Take a moment to answer these questions:
What details most helped me recognize the conflict of the folk tale?

How could I apply the message of this story to modern life?

Have you ever wished you could do something that you knew was physically impossible?

Reach Into Your Background

Even though we really can't do it, we sometimes imagine what it might be like to expand our physical powers. You might imagine being able to fly above your home or school, or swim underwater for long periods of time without having to come up for air. What if you could function without sleep?

Be careful! Don't try out any of these flights of fancy because they all involve serious dangers. You can, however, let your imagination soar safely as you complete one or both of the following activities:

- Write about an impossible wish you have had about physical powers. Use vivid details to describe what the experience would be like.
- With a partner, list the positive and negative aspects of such a wish.

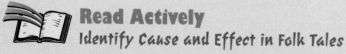

Read Actively
Identify Cause and Effect in Folk Tales

When you imagine yourself in impossible situations, you may not always think about the consequences of these wishes. You'd see a lot more if you stopped to consider the **effects,** or results, of any actions you take. From the safe environment of a reader's armchair, folk tales often give readers an opportunity to learn about **causes,** what makes something happen, and their sometimes dangerous effects.

In this folk tale a young boy wants to do something that he knows will cause him great harm. As you read, look for the cause of his wish and the effects it has on him and his family.

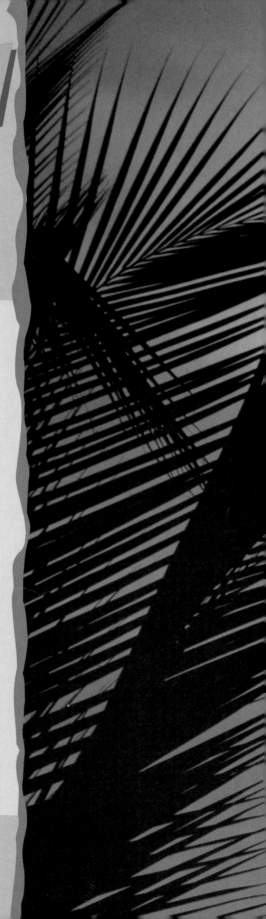

CHILDREN of WAX

from Zimbabwe

Alexander McCall Smith

Not far from the hills of the Matopos[1] there lived a family whose children were made out of wax. The mother and the father in this family were exactly the same as everyone else, but for some reason their children had turned out to be made of wax. At first this caused them great sorrow, and they wondered who had put such a spell on them, but later they became quite accustomed to this state of affairs and grew to love their children dearly.

It was easy for the parents to love the wax children. While other children might fight among themselves or forget to do their duty, wax children were always dutiful and never fought with one another. They were also hard workers, one wax child being able to do the work of at least two ordinary children.

Mask topped by a bird Yaore people
Ivory Coast Art Resource, New York, New York

---

1. the hills of the Matopos (mah TOH pohz): The blue granite mountains of Matabeleland (mat uh BEE lee land), a part of Zimbabwe (zim BAH bway) in eastern Africa.

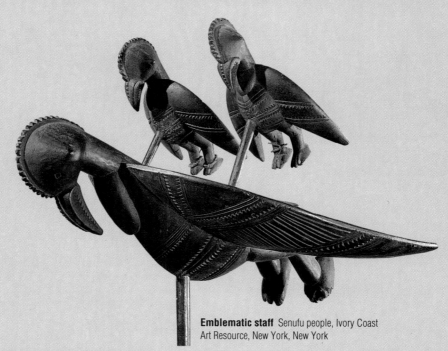

Emblematic staff Senufu people, Ivory Coast
Art Resource, New York, New York

The only real problem which the wax children gave was that people had to avoid making fires too close to them, and of course they also had to work only at night. If they worked during the day, when the sun was hot, wax children would melt.

To keep them out of the sun, their father made the wax children a dark hut that had no windows. During the day no rays of the sun could penetrate into the gloom of this hut, and so the wax children were quite safe. Then, when the sun had gone down, the children would come out of their dark hut and begin their work. They tended the crops and watched over the cattle, just as ordinary children did during the daytime.

There was one wax child, Ngwabi,[2] who used to talk about what it was like during the day.

"We can never know what the world is like," he said to his brothers and sisters. "When we come out of our hut everything is quite dark and we see so little."

Ngwabi's brothers and sisters knew that what he said was right, but they accepted they would never know what the world looked like. There were other things that they had which the other children did not have, and

they contented themselves with these. They knew, for instance, that other children felt pain: wax children never experienced pain, and for this they were grateful.

But poor Ngwabi still longed to see the world. In his dreams he saw the hills in the distance and watched the clouds that brought rain. He saw paths that led this way and that through the bush, and he longed to be able to follow them. But that was something that a wax child could never do, as it was far too dangerous to follow such paths in the night-time.

As he grew older, this desire of Ngwabi's to see what the world was really like when the sun was up grew stronger and stronger. At last he was unable to contain it any more and he ran out of the hut one day when the sun was riding high in the sky and all about there was light and more light. The other children screamed, and some of them tried to grab at him as he left the hut, but they failed to stop their brother and he was gone.

Words to Know

penetrate (PEN uh trayt) v.: Pass into or through
contented (kuhn TENT id) v.: Satisfied
peering (PEER ing) v.: Looking closely

---

2. Ngwabi (en GWAH bee)

Of course he could not last long in such heat. The sun burned down on Ngwabi and before he had taken more than a few steps he felt all the strength drain from his limbs. Crying out to his brothers and sisters, he fell to the ground and was soon nothing more that a pool of wax in the dust. Inside the hut, afraid to leave its darkness, the other wax children wept for their melted brother.

When night came, the children left their hut and went to the spot where Ngwabi had fallen. Picking up the wax, they went to a special place they knew and there Ngwabi's eldest sister made the wax into a bird. It was a bird with great wings and for feathers they put a covering or leaves from the trees that grew there. These leaves would protect the wax from the sun so that it would not melt when it became day.

After they had finished their task, they told their parents what had happened. The man and woman wept, and each of them kissed the wax model of a bird. Then they set it upon a rock that stood before the wax children's hut.

The wax children did not work that night. At dawn, they were all in their hut, peering through a small crack that there was in the wall. As the light came up over the hills, it made the wax bird seem pink with fire. Then, as the sun itself rose over the fields, the great bird which they had made suddenly moved its wings and launched itself into the air. Soon it was high above the ground, circling over the children's hut. A few minutes later it was gone, and the children knew that their brother was happy at last.

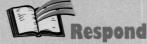

Respond

- Do you think Ngwabi made a wise decision? Why?
- With a partner, describe the events you could add to create a happier ending. What events would create a sadder one?

Alexander McCall Smith was born and raised in Zimbabwe, a country in south-central Africa. He has traveled widely throughout that country gathering its folklore. In addition to "Children of Wax," Smith has collected stories from both children and older people.

The land of **Zimbabwe** and the countries surrounding it once held civilizations that thrived a thousand years ago. Since that era, most of sub-Saharan Africa has been populated by tribal communities whose people survive by farming, hunting, fishing, or herding. The land is rich and supports a variety of plant and animal life. However, drought, famine, disease, and predatory animals can make the region dangerous. In the face of these hazards, many African folk tales stress the importance of family and community ties.

Explore Your Reading
Look Back (Recall)

1. How do the lives of the wax children differ from those of other children?
2. How is Ngwabi different from his siblings?

Think It Over (Interpret)

3. What details about the children could be true only in fantasy?
4. What is realistic about them?

Go Beyond (Apply)

5. Could a real child be content with the kind of life that the wax children had? Explain.

Develop Reading and Literary Skills
Understand Metamorphosis in a Folk Tale

You probably noticed that Ngwabi's dreams caused great danger. This folk tale would be much different if he were to meet his end as a puddle of wax. Instead, the boy experiences a **metamorphosis,** a complete change of form. His brothers and sisters help reshape him into something else and he continues to live.

Some folk tales and myths use metamorphosis to punish characters for bad behavior. One well known folk tale, for example, explains how King Midas turns his daughter into a gold statue when his greed takes over his common sense.

To understand Ngwabi's metamorphosis and its meaning, you should consider how it occurs. His desire for freedom causes him to run out into the sun's heat. Consider the following questions:

1. What do Ngwabi's siblings do after he melts into a pool of wax?
2. What is unusual about the way the bird comes to life?
3. What happens to the bird at the end?
4. How is the ending appropriate?

Ideas for Writing

In "Children of Wax," children could be made of wax and changed into flying birds. In fantasy, anything can happen.

Fantasy Create your own fantastic characters and the world in which they live. Use real and imaginary details to write a brief fantasy featuring the characters you imagined.

Character's Farewell Imagine Ngwabi has been granted a wish to become human for exactly one hour. Write the letter he might send to his family. Include the cause and effect of Ngwabi's actions, details of his new life, and assurances that he is okay.

Ideas for Projects

Landscape Create a drawing or three-dimensional model to show the kinds of things Ngwabi and his siblings never got the chance to see. You can add descriptions to your illustration that explain the features of the Zimbabwe landscape. [Art Link]

Weather Report Research the heat in Harare, Zimbabwe's capital city. Prepare a chart that compares the average monthly temperatures there with a city near you. Explain the causes and effects of the weather in each city. Draw conclusions from your comparison and give reasons for the differences in temperature. [Science Link; Math Link]

How Am I Doing?

Respond to these questions in your journal:

What did I find easy about identifying cause and effect? What did I find difficult?

How could a knowledge of cause-and-effect-relationships help me study history or science?

What Is My Responsibility to Others?

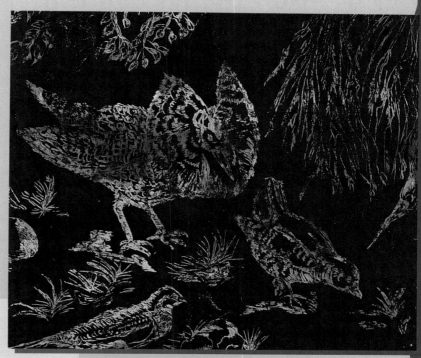

Student Art ***Three Birds*** Judit Santak
Hungary, Paintbrush Diplomacy

Spring

Student Writing Emma Greig
Rochester, Michigan

It's time for birth and life.
and death?
I hear calls from the flashes of iridescent
amethyst soaring above my head.
Something is not right
something is out of place.
A hatchling purple martin
has fallen
from the
colony bird house.
Pink and helpless
no chance for life.
Or is there?
Should I aid the fallen chick?
Or trust in nature's ways?

I walked away.

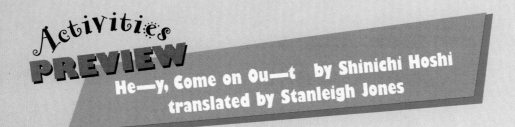

Activities
PREVIEW
He—y, Come on Ou—t by Shinichi Hoshi
translated by Stanleigh Jones

How will your choices affect future generations?

Reach Into Your Background

Many of the environmental problems of today resulted from the choices of yesterday. For example, hazardous waste sites built up as corporations and governments added to them bit by bit. Now we're more aware that today's choices shape tomorrow's world.

In a group, do one or both of these activities to explore the consequences of our decisions:

- Sketch out a chart to show how a choice made years ago affects you today. For example, consider the choice in the 1950's to build many interstate highways.
- Role-play a television newscast from the year 2150. Show how some environmental problems result from choices made fifty years earlier.

Read Actively
Make Predictions About a Story

Writers of science fiction often make **predictions,** or educated guesses, about the the future. In reading, too, you can make predictions about a story's ending. You can base these on what characters do, think, and say, and on your own experience. For example, if polluting the environment leads to trouble in real life, it may cause the same result in fiction. By making predictions, you will become more involved with a story.

As you read this science-fiction story, jot down clues to the ending. Look for what characters do or fail to do, and remember what you know about the consequences of decisions. Then use your clues to make predictions about what will happen.

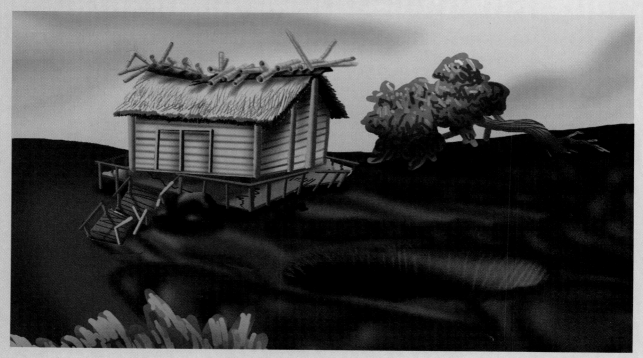

Illustration by Everett Magie

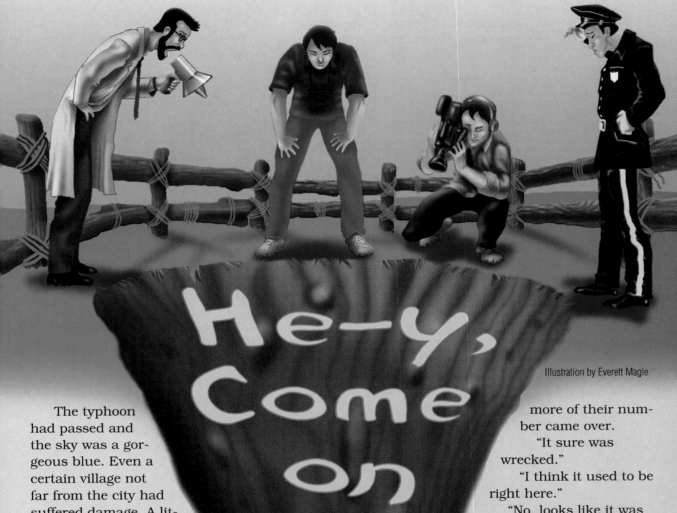

Illustration by Everett Magie

He—y, Come on Ou—t!

Shinichi Hoshi
translated by Stanleigh Jones

The typhoon had passed and the sky was a gorgeous blue. Even a certain village not far from the city had suffered damage. A little distance from the village and near the mountains, a small shrine had been swept away by a landslide.

"I wonder how long that shrine's been here."

"Well, in any case, it must have been here since an awfully long time ago."

"We've got to rebuild it right away."

While the villagers exchanged views, several more of their number came over.

"It sure was wrecked."

"I think it used to be right here."

"No, looks like it was a little more over there."

Just then one of them raised his voice. "Hey what in the world is this hole?"

Where they had all gathered there was a hole about a meter in diameter. They peered in, but it was so dark nothing could be seen. However, it gave one the feeling that it was so deep it went clear through to the center of the earth.

There was even one person who said, "I wonder if it's a fox's hole."

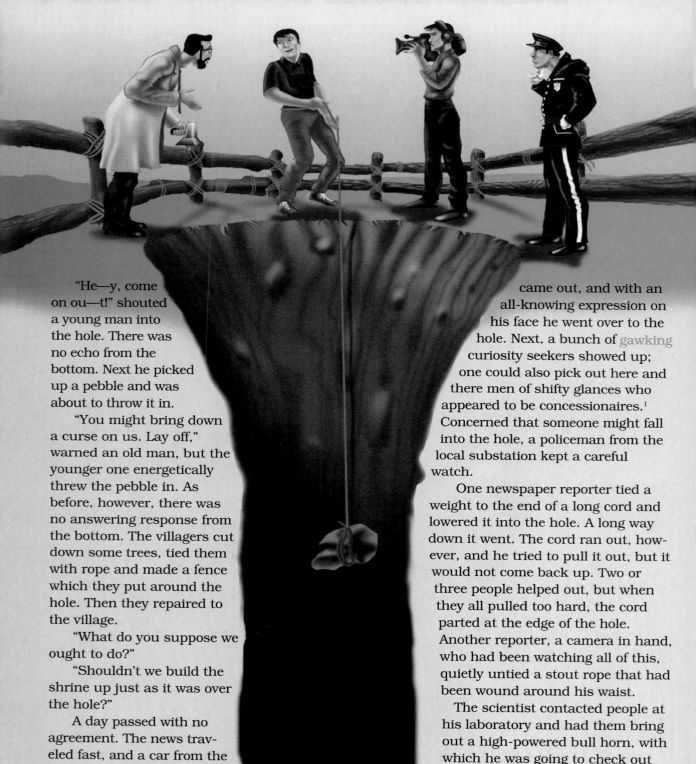

"He—y, come on ou—t!" shouted a young man into the hole. There was no echo from the bottom. Next he picked up a pebble and was about to throw it in.

"You might bring down a curse on us. Lay off," warned an old man, but the younger one energetically threw the pebble in. As before, however, there was no answering response from the bottom. The villagers cut down some trees, tied them with rope and made a fence which they put around the hole. Then they repaired to the village.

"What do you suppose we ought to do?"

"Shouldn't we build the shrine up just as it was over the hole?"

A day passed with no agreement. The news traveled fast, and a car from the newspaper company rushed over. In no time a scientist

came out, and with an all-knowing expression on his face he went over to the hole. Next, a bunch of gawking curiosity seekers showed up; one could also pick out here and there men of shifty glances who appeared to be concessionaires.[1] Concerned that someone might fall into the hole, a policeman from the local substation kept a careful watch.

One newspaper reporter tied a weight to the end of a long cord and lowered it into the hole. A long way down it went. The cord ran out, however, and he tried to pull it out, but it would not come back up. Two or three people helped out, but when they all pulled too hard, the cord parted at the edge of the hole. Another reporter, a camera in hand, who had been watching all of this, quietly untied a stout rope that had been wound around his waist.

The scientist contacted people at his laboratory and had them bring out a high-powered bull horn, with which he was going to check out the echo from the hole's bottom. He tried switching through various sounds, but there was no echo. The scientist was puzzled, but he could

1. **concessionaires** (kuhn sesh uh NAYRZ) *n.*: Business people.

Illustration by Everett Magie

not very well give up with everyone watching him so intently. He put the bull horn right up to the hole, turned it to its highest volume, and let it sound continuously for a long time. It was a noise that would have carried several dozen kilometers above ground. But the hole just calmly swallowed up the sound.

In his own mind the scientist was at a loss, but with a look of apparent composure he cut off the sound and, in a manner suggesting that the whole thing had a perfectly plausible explanation, said simply, "Fill it in."

Safer to get rid of something one didn't understand.

The onlookers, disappointed that this was all that was going to happen, prepared to disperse. Just then one of the concessionaires, having broken through the throng and come forward, made a proposal.

"Let me have that hole. I'll fill it in for you."

"We'd be grateful to you for filling it in," replied the mayor of the village, "but we can't very well give you the hole. We have to build a shrine there."

"If it's a shrine you want, I'll build you a fine one later. Shall I make it with an attached meeting hall?"

Before the mayor could answer, the people of the village all shouted out.

"Really? Well, in that case, we ought to have it closer to the village."

"It's just an old hole. We'll give it to you!"

So it was settled. And the mayor, of course, had no objection.

The concessionaire was true to his promise. It was small, but closer to the village he did build for them a shrine with an attached meeting hall.

About the time the autumn festival was held at the new shrine, the hole-filling company established by the concessionaire hung out its small shingle at a shack near the hole.

The concessionaire had his cohorts mount a loud campaign in the city. "We've got a fabulously deep hole! Scientists say it's at least five thousand meters deep! Perfect for the disposal of such things as waste from nuclear reactors."

Government authorities granted permission. Nuclear power plants fought for contracts. The people of the village were a bit worried about this, but they consented when it was explained that there would be absolutely no above-ground contamination[2] for several thousand years and that they would share in the profits. Into the bargain, very shortly a magnificent road was built from the city to the village.

Trucks rolled in over the road, transporting lead boxes. Above the hole the lids were opened, and the wastes from nuclear reactors tumbled away into the hole.

From the Foreign Ministry and the Defense Agency boxes of unnecessary classified documents[3] were brought for disposal.

---

2. **contamination** (kuhn tam i NAY shun) n.: Pollution by poison or other dangerous substances.

3. **classified documents:** Secret government papers.

Illustration by Everett Magie

Officials who came to supervise the disposal held discussions on golf. The lesser functionaries, as they threw in the papers, chatted about pinball.

The hole showed no signs of filling up. It was awfully deep, thought some; or else it might be very spacious at the bottom. Little by little the hole-filling company expanded its business.

Bodies of animals used in contagious disease experiments at the universities were brought out, and to these were added the unclaimed corpses of vagrants. Better than dumping all of its garbage in the ocean, went the thinking in the city, and plans were made for a long pipe to carry it to the hole.

The hole gave peace of mind to the dwellers of the city. They concentrated solely on producing one thing after another. Everyone disliked thinking about the eventual consequences. People wanted only to work for production companies and sales corporations; they had no interest in becoming junk dealers. But, it was thought, these problems too would gradually be resolved by the hole.

Young girls whose betrothals[4] had been arranged discarded old diaries in the hole. There were also those who were inaugurating new love affairs and threw into the hole old photographs of themselves taken with former sweethearts. The police felt comforted as they used the hole to get rid of accumulations of expertly done counterfeit bills. Criminals breathed easier after throwing material evidence into the hole.

Whatever one wished to discard, the hole accepted it all. The hole cleansed the city of its filth; the sea and sky seemed to have become a bit clearer than before.

Aiming at the heavens, new buildings went on being constructed one after the other.

One day, atop the high steel frame of a new building under construction, a workman was taking a break. Above his head he heard a voice shout:

"He—y, come on ou—t!"

---

4. betrothals (bee TROH thuhlz) *n.*: Engagements to be married.

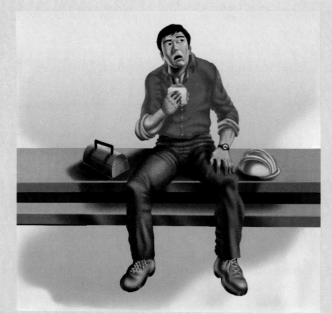

Illustration by Everett Magie

But, in the sky to which he lifted his gaze there was nothing at all. A clear blue sky merely spread over all. He thought it must be his imagination. Then, as he resumed his former position, from the direction where the voice had come, a small pebble skimmed by him and fell on past.

The man, however, was gazing in idle reverie[5] at the city's skyline growing ever more beautiful, and he failed to notice.

---

5. idle reverie (REV uh ree): Daydreaming.

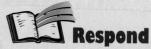 **Respond**

- Were you surprised by the ending? Why or why not?
- With a small group, compare and contrast this science-fiction story with real life. Jot down some details that are realistic and some that aren't.

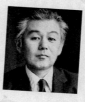

Shinichi Hoshi
(SHIH NEE SHEE HOH SHEE) (1926–   ) is a Japanese author famous for his award-winning science-fiction stories.

MAKE MEANING

Explore Your Reading

Look Back (Recall)

1. How do people react to and use the hole?

Think It Over (Interpret)

2. Why does the concessionaire want the hole?
3. How does the hole give everyone "peace of mind"?
4. What is actually happening at the end of the story?
5. What is the theme, or central idea, of this story?

Go Beyond (Apply)

6. Would you want the characters in this story to live near you? Explain your answer.

Develop Reading and Literary Skills

Appreciate a Surprise Ending

You may not have predicted the ending of this story. That's because Hoshi wrote a **surprise ending,** a conclusion with an unexpected twist. When you go back over the story, however, you will find hints to the surprise. One hint, for example, is the old man's warning at the beginning of the story. He fears that throwing something into the hole may "bring down a curse on us."

Writers can use a surprise ending to underline a point. By giving readers a shock, they can make them think about their own behavior.

1. Find another hint to the surprise ending, and explain your choice.
2. Why is the ending a shock?
3. What does the writer want to shock you into doing?

Ideas for Writing

Hoshi points out that the choices we make today affect future generations.

TV Feature Story Imagine that you are a television newswriter living in 2150. Write a feature story for a news program showing how past decisions affect your world.

Science-Fiction Story Write a science-fiction story to show how today's choices will affect tomorrow's world. Like Shinichi Hoshi, combine realistic details with imaginary ones. You might even consider using a surprise ending.

Ideas for Projects

Video/Computer Game Design a computer or video game that helps young people to see the effects of environmental choices. Give rewards for wise choices and penalties for foolish ones. Share your game with classmates. [Science Link]

Poster Campaign Create a series of posters to educate others about environmental issues. For example, your posters could encourage recycling and discourage littering and waste. Get the permission of your principal to display your posters throughout the school. [Science Link; Art Link]

Speaker From the Community Invite a speaker from an organization that is concerned about the environment. Ask the person to talk to your class about environmental issues, and have students prepare their own questions. [Science Link]

How Am I Doing?

Answer these questions to evaluate how well you're doing:

What did I learn about making predictions as I read? How could I use this skill with other types of reading?

Which example of my work will I put in my portfolio? Why?

What do animals think of us?

Reach Into Your Background

All of us tend to think that human errands are far more important than animal errands, whatever they may be. However, it's interesting to imagine how we might seem to an ant, for instance, as we go about our important business. From the ant's-eye view, we might look like a tower of a creature, a walking earthquake, or a traveling disaster.

Do one or both of these activities to continue thinking about the way animals look at us:

- In a group, discuss books you've read or movies you've seen that show the world from an animal's point of view.
- As a particular kind of animal, deliver a speech about humans and human activities from your point of view.

Read Actively
Visualize Images in Poetry

Viewing humans from an animal's point of view probably called up vivid **images,** or pictures, in your mind. Poets often use images to help you see and experience the world in a livelier way. These images appeal not only to your sense of sight, but also to your senses of touch, taste, smell, and hearing. By **visualizing,** or letting yourself experience, images in poetry, you will see the world in a fresh way.

Find the images in these poems, and to help you visualize them, fill in a chart like this as you read.

Poem	Image	Senses
The Bait	"damp California grass"	sight and touch

The Bait

Eric Chock

Saturday mornings, before
my weekly chores,
I used to sneak out of the house
and across the street,
5   grabbing the first grasshopper
waking in the damp California grass
along the stream.
Carefully hiding a silver hook
beneath its green wings,
10 I'd float it out
across the gentle ripples
towards the end of its life.
Just like that.
I'd give it the hook
15 and let it ride.
All I ever expected for it
was that big-mouth bass
awaiting its arrival.
I didn't think
20 that I was giving up one life
to get another,
that even childhood
was full of sacrifice.
I'd just take the bright green thing,
25 pluck it off its only stalk,
and give it away as if
it were mine to give.
I knew someone out there
would be fooled,
30 that someone would accept
the precious gift.
So I just sent it along
with a plea of a prayer,
hoping it would spread its wings this time
35 and fly across that wet glass sky,
no concern for what inspired
its life, or mine,
only instinct guiding pain
towards the other side.

Eric Chock (1950–   ) is the coordinator of the Hawaii Poets in the Schools program, which brings local poets into public schools. Chock believes that when Hawaiian students begin learning about the literature of their own culture, they will feel "more pride . . . and an awareness of Hawaii's past and present."

Words to Know

sacrifice (SAK ruh fīs) n.: Loss; giving up one thing for the sake of something else (line 23)
instinct (IN stinkt) n.: A way of acting that is natural to people and animals from birth, not learned (line 38)

Birdfoot's Grampa

Joseph Bruchac

The Old Man
must have stopped our car
two dozen times to climb out
and gather into his hands
5   the small toads blinded
by our lights and leaping
like live drops of rain.

The rain was falling,
a mist around his white hair,
10 and I kept saying,
"You can't save them all,
accept it, get in,
we've got places to go."

But, leathery hands full
15 of wet brown life,
knee deep in the summer
roadside grass,
he just smiled and said,
"They have places to go, too."

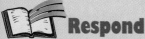

Respond

- Which images from these poems stay in your mind? Why?
- In a small group, discuss whether or not these poems made you think differently about your experiences with animals.

Joseph Bruchac (1942–   ) says, "When an African carver takes a branch from a tree to shape it into a mask, he first asks permission from the spirit of that tree. When an Iroquois healer gathers herbs, she places tobacco on the Earth in exchange. It is important to keep the balance."

MAKE MEANING

Explore Your Reading

Look Back (Recall)

1. What takes place between animals and humans in each poem?

Think It Over (Interpret)

2. As a boy, how did the speaker in "The Bait" feel about using grasshoppers as bait?
3. As an adult, does he feel the same way? Explain.
4. What idea is the Old Man trying to teach in "Birdfoot's Grampa"?
5. In what way is the speaker of each poem criticizing himself?

Go Beyond (Apply)

6. What might happen if the Old Man from "Birdfoot's Grampa" met the boy from "The Bait"? Explain.

Develop Reading and Literary Skills

Examine Images in Poetry

You've probably noted many of the **images,** or pictures, in these poems. Poets create images by using language that appeals to all your senses. For example, in "The Bait," Chock remembers "grabbing the first grasshopper / waking in the damp California grass." This image appeals to your senses of sight and touch, and you can almost feel yourself reaching for the grasshopper.

Besides being lively in themselves, images can help a poet get a point across. In these poems, the images make the animals seem vivid, fragile, and "precious." As a result, you may be more willing to look at things from their point of view.

1. In each of these poems, find an image that makes an animal seem more alive. Explain your choices.
2. Find a sense that is ignored in the images from these poems. Then create an image for each poem that appeals to this sense.

Ideas for Writing

Imagery plays an important role not only in poetry but in other forms of writing as well.

Poem As an animal, write a poem that describes an encounter with a human being. You might even want to write as one of Bruchac's toads or Chock's grasshoppers. Use vivid images to express your feelings and ideas.

Letter to the Editor Humane treatment of animals is a subject that many people feel strongly about. Write a letter to your local or school paper that expresses your opinions on this issue. Support your points with images, as well as examples and facts.

Ideas for Projects

Zoo Report Find out how modern zoos are trying to treat animals in a kinder fashion. Present your results to your classmates in an oral report. If possible, illustrate your talk with pictures or even videotapes of the zoos you are discussing. [Science Link]

Annotated Movie Guide Prepare a guide that contains brief reviews of movies featuring animals. Note how well the animals seem to be treated, and suggest who should see the films. You might want to develop a rating system such as a four-paw mark for excellent and a three-paw mark for good.

How Am I Doing?

Respond to these questions in your journal:
How did understanding imagery help me to appreciate these poems better? What could I do to improve my understanding of images in poetry?

How did reading poems about animals help me understand how our choices affect others?

When have you reached out to help a plant, an animal, a person?

Reach Into Your Background

The plant in your living room has a woeful look and one of its leaves is shriveling. A stray cat, a calico, has been wandering your block, pressing close to the buildings and meowing deeply from its belly. A friend who's moving to another city pats you on the shoulder and asks for help with the packing . . . What do you owe to others in need?

Think about this question as you do one or both of these activities:

*   Go over the events of a recent week and jot down the times when your help was needed in some way.
*   Tell a partner a story about a time when you reached out to help someone or something.

Read Actively
Gather Evidence About Symbols

Organizations that help people sometimes have **symbols,** like a red cross, that stand for what they do. Symbols help in communication because they sum up complicated ideas and feelings. That's why writers use symbols in stories. Something ordinary, like a bird, can stand for more than it usually does. By gathering evidence about symbols, you'll be tuning in to a writer's meanings.

In "Power," a trapped bird and a power line are symbols. As you read the story, look for passages that hint at their meaning. Write your ideas in a chart like this one.

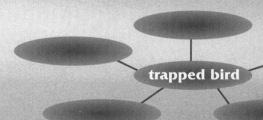

trapped bird

power line

Power

Jack Cope

From the gum tree at the corner he looked out over, well—nothing. There was nothing more after his father's place, only the veld,[1] so flat and unchanging that the single shadowy koppie[2] away off towards the skyline made it look more empty still. It was a lonely koppie like himself.

The one thing that made a difference was the powerline. High above the earth on its giant steel lattice towers, the powerline strode across the veld until it disappeared beyond the koppie. It passed close to his father's place and one of the great pylons was on their ground in a square patch fenced off with barbed wire, a forbidden place. André used to look through the wire at the pylon. Around the steelwork itself were more screens of barbed wire, and on all four sides of it enamel warning-plates with a red skull-and-crossbones said in three languages, DANGER! And there was a huge figure of volts, millions of volts.

André was ten and he knew volts were electricity and the line took power by a short cut far across country. It worked gold mines, it lit towns, and hauled trains and drove machinery somewhere out beyond. The power station was in the town ten miles on the other side of his father's place and the great line simply jumped right over them without stopping.

André filled the empty spaces in his life by imagining things. Often he was a jet plane and roared around the house and along the paths with his arms outspread. He saw an Everest film once and for a long time he was Hillary or Tensing,[3] or both, conquering a mountain. There were no mountains so he conquered the roof of the house which wasn't very high and was made of red-painted tin. But he reached the summit and planted a flag on the lightning conductor. When he got down his mother hit his legs with a quince switch for being naughty.

Another time he conquered the koppie. It took him the whole afternoon to get there and back and it was not as exciting as he expected, being less steep than it looked from a distance, so he did not need his rope and pick. Also, he found a cow had beaten him to the summit.

He thought of conquering one of the powerline towers. It had everything, the danger especially, and studying it from all

---

1. veld (VELT) *n.*: Open grassy country with few bushes and almost no trees.

2. koppie (KAHP ee) *n.*: In South Africa, a small hill.

3. Hillary (HIL uhr ee) **or Tensing** (TEN zing): Sir Edmund Hillary and Tensing Norgay, the first two men to climb to the top of Mt. Everest and return.

Words to Know

lattice (LAT uhs) *n.*: A structure of crossed strips of wood or metal, used as a support

pylons (PĪ lahnz) *n.*: Towerlike structures

summit (SUHM it) *n.*: The highest point; the top

sides he guessed he could make the summit without touching a live wire.[4] But he was not as disobedient as all that, and he knew if he so much as went inside the barbed-wire fence his mother would skin him with the quince, not to mention his father. There were peaks which had to remain unconquered.

He used to lie and listen to the marvelous hum of the power-line, the millions of volts flowing invisible and beyond all one's ideas along the copper wires that hung so smooth and light from ties of crinkled white china looking like chinese lanterns up against the sky. Faint cracklings and murmurs and rushes of sound would sometimes come from the powerline, and at night he was sure he saw soft blue flames lapping and trembling on the wires as if they were only half peeping out of that fierce river of volts. The flames danced and their voices chattered to him of a mystery.

In the early morning when the mist was rising and the first sun's rays were shooting underneath it, the powerline sparkled like a tremendous spiderweb. It took his thoughts away into a magical distance, far—far off among gigantic machines and busy factories. That was where the world opened up. So he loved the powerline dearly. It made a door through the distance for his thoughts. It was like him except that it never slept, and while he was dreaming it went on without stopping, crackling faintly and murmuring. Its electricity hauled up the mine skips[5] from the heart of the earth, hurtled huge green rail units along their shining lines, and thundered day and night in the factories.

Now that the veld's green was darkening and gathering black-and-gold tints from the ripe seeds and withering grass blades, now that clear warm autumn days were coming after the summer thunderstorms, the birds began gathering on the powerline. At evening he would see the wires like necklaces of blue-and-black glass beads when the swallows gathered. It took them days and days, it seemed, to make up their minds. He did not know whether the same swallows collected each evening in growing numbers or whether a batch went off each day to be replaced by others. He did not know enough about them. He loved to hear them making excited twittering sounds, he loved to see how they simply fell off the copper wire into space and their perfect curved wings lifted them on the air.

They were going not merely beyond the skyline like the power, they were flying thousands of miles over land and sea and moun-tains and forests to countries he had never dreamed of. They would fly over Everest, perhaps, they would see ships below them

---

4. live wire: A wire with electricity running through it, which is potentially dangerous to touch.

5. mine skips: Small, open carts in which miners and materials travel up and down mine shafts.

on blue seas among islands, they would build nests under bridges and on chimneys where other boys in funny clothes would watch them. The birds opened another door for him and he liked them too, very much.

He watched the swallows one morning as they took off from their perch. Suddenly, as if they had a secret signal, a whole stretch of them along a wire would start together. They dropped forward into the air and their blue-and-white wings flicked out. Flying seemed to be the easiest thing in the world. They swooped and flew up, crisscrossing in flight and chirping crazily, so pleased to be awake in the morning. Then another flight of them winged off, and another. There was standing-room only on those wires. Close to the lofty pylon and the gleaming china ties another flight took off. But one of the swallows stayed behind, quite close to the tie. André watched them fall forward, but it alone did not leave the line. It flapped its wings and he saw it was caught by its leg.

He should have been going to school but he stood watching the swallow, his cap pulled over his white hair and eyes wrinkled against the light. After a minute the swallow stopped flapping and hung there. He wondered how it could have got caught, maybe in the wire binding or at a join. Swallows had short legs and small black claws; he had caught one once in its nest and held it in his hands before it struggled free and was gone in a flash. He thought the bird on the power-line would get free soon, but looking at it there he had a tingling kind of pain in his chest and in one leg as if he too were caught by the foot. André wanted to rush back and tell his mother, only she would scold him for being late to school. So he climbed on his bike, and with one more look up at the helpless bird there against the sky and the steel framework of the tower, he rode off to the bus.

At school he thought once or twice about the swallow, but mostly he forgot about it and that made him feel bad. Anyway, he thought, it would be free by the time he got home. Twisting and flapping a few times, it was sure to work its foot out; and there was no need for him to worry about it hanging there.

"Couldn't—?" he began.

"Couldn't nothing, dear," she said quite firmly so that he knew she meant business. "Now stop thinking about it, and tomorrow you'll see."

His father came home at six and had tea, and afterwards there was a little time to work in his patch of vegetables out at the back. André followed him and he soon got round to the swallow on the powerline.

"I know," his father said. "Mama told me."

"It's still there."

"Well—" his father tilted up his old working-hat and looked at him hard with his sharp blue eyes "—well, we can't do anything about it, can we, now?"

"No, Papa, but—"

"But what?"

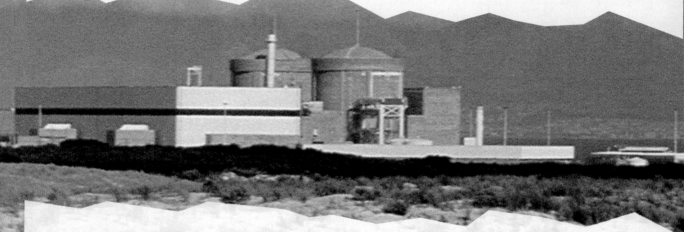

Coming back from the crossroads he felt anxious, but he did not like to look up until he was quite near. Then he shot one glance at the top of the pylon—the swallow was still there, its wings spread but not moving. It was dead, he guessed, as he stopped and put down one foot. Then he saw it flutter and fold up its wings. He felt awful to think it had hung there all day, trapped. The boy went in and called his mother and they stood off some distance below the powerline and looked at the bird. The mother shaded her eyes with her hand. It was a pity, she said, but really she was sure it would free itself somehow. Nothing could be done about it.

He kicked at a stone, and said nothing more. He could see his father was kind of stiff about it; that meant he did not want to hear anything more. They had been talking about it, and maybe—yes, that was it. They were afraid he would try to climb up the pylon.

At supper none of them talked about the swallow, but André felt it all right. He felt as if it was hanging above their heads and his mother and father felt it and they all had a load on them. Going to bed his mother said to him he must not worry himself about the poor bird. "Not a sparrow falls without our Good Lord knowing."

"It's not a sparrow, it's a swallow," he said. "It's going to hang there all night, by its foot." His mother sighed and put out the light. She was worried.

The next day was a Saturday and he did not have to go to school. First thing he looked out and the bird was still there. The other swallows were with it, and when they took off it fluttered and made little thin calls but could not get free.

He would rather have been at school instead of knowing all day that it was hanging up there on the cruel wire. It was strange how the electricity did nothing to it. He knew, of course, that the wires were quite safe as long as you did not touch anything else. The morning was very long, though he did forget about the swallow quite often. He was building a mud fort under the gum tree, and he had to carry water and dig up the red earth and mix it into a stiff clay. When he was coming in at midday with his khaki hat flapping round his face he had one more look and what he saw kept him standing there a long time with his mouth open. Other swallows were fluttering and hovering around the trapped bird, trying to help it. He rushed inside and dragged his mother out by her hand and she stood too, shading her eyes again and looking up.

"Yes, they're feeding it. Isn't that strange," she said.

"Sssh! Don't frighten them," he whispered.

In the afternoon he lay in the grass and twice again he saw the other swallows fluttering round the fastened bird with short quivering strokes of their wings and opening their beaks wide. Swallows had pouches in their throats where they made small mud bricks to build their nests, and that was how they brought food to it. They knew how to feed their fledglings[6] and when the trapped bird squeaked and cried out they brought it food. André felt choked thinking how they helped it and nobody else would do anything. His parents would not even talk about it.

---

6. **fledglings** (FLEJ lingz) *n.*: Young birds that have just grown the feathers needed for flying.

With his keen eyes he traced the way a climber could get up the tower. Most difficult would be to get round the barbed-wire screens about a quarter of the way up. After that there were footholds in the steel lattice supports. He had studied it before. But if you did get up, what then? How could you touch the swallow? Just putting your hand near the wire, wouldn't those millions of volts flame out and jump at you? The only thing was to get somebody to turn off the power for a minute, then he could whip up the tower like a monkey. At supper that night he suggested it, and his father was as grim and angry as he'd ever been.

"Crumbs," André said to himself. "Crumbs! They are both het up about it."

"Listen, son," his father had said. He never said "son" unless he was really mad over something. "Listen, I don't want you to get all worked up about that bird. I'll see what can be done. But you leave it alone. Don't get any ideas into your head, and don't go near that pylon."

"What ideas, Papa?" he asked, trembling inside himself.

"Any ideas at all."

"The other birds are feeding it, but it may die."

"Well, I'm sorry; try not to think about it."

When his mother came to say goodnight to him he turned his face over into his pillow and would not kiss her. It was something he had never done before and it was because he was angry with them both. They let the swallow swing there in the night and did nothing.

His mother patted his back and ruffled his white hair and said, "Goodnight, darling." But he gritted his teeth and did not answer.

Ages seemed to him to have passed. On Sunday the bird was still hanging on the lofty powerline, fluttering feebly. He could not bear to look up at it. After breakfast he went out and tried to carry on building his fort under the gum tree. The birds were chattering in the tree above him and in the wattles[7] at the back of the house. Through the corner of his eye he saw a handsome black-and-white bird fly out in swinging loops from the tree and it settled on the powerline some distance from the tower. It was a butcher-bird, a Jackey-hangman, a terrible greedy pirate of a bird. His heart fell like a stone—he just guessed what it was up to. It sat there on the wire impudently copying the calls of other birds. It could imitate a toppie or a robin or a finch as it liked. It stole their naked little kickers from their nests and spiked them on the barbed wire to eat at pleasure, as it stole their songs too. The butcher-bird flew off and settled higher up the wire near the pylon.

André rushed up the path and then took a swing from the house to come under the powerline. Stopping, he saw the other birds were making a whirl and fluttered round the cannibal. Swallows darted and skimmed and made him duck his head, but he went on sitting there. Then some starlings came screaming out of the gum tree and flew in a menacing bunch at the butcher-bird. They all hated him. He made the mistake of losing his balance and fluttered out into the air and all the birds were round him at once, darting and pecking and screaming.

The butcher-bird pulled off one of his typical tricks: he fell plumb down and when near the ground spread his wings, sailed low over the shrubs, and came up at the house where he settled on the lightning conductor. André stood panting and felt his heart beating fast. He wanted to throw a stone at the butcher-bird but he reckoned the stone would land on the roof and get him in trouble. So he ran towards the house waving his arms and shouting. The bird cocked its head and watched him.

---

7. **wattles** (WAHT uhlz) *n.*: Frameworks or piles of sticks, branches, etc.

His mother came out. "Darling, what's the matter?"

"That Jackey, he's on the roof. He wanted to kill the swallow."

"Oh, darling!" the mother said softly.

It was Sunday night and he said to his mother, "It's only the other birds keeping him alive. They were feeding him again today."

"I saw them."

"He can't live much longer, Mama. And now the Jackey knows he's there. Why can't Papa get them to switch off the electricity?"

"They wouldn't do it for a bird, darling. Now try and go to sleep."

Leaving for school on Monday, he tried not to look up. But he couldn't help it and there was the swallow spreading and closing its wings. He quickly got on his bike and rode as fast as he could. He could not think of anything but the trapped bird on the powerline.

After school, André did not catch the bus home. Instead he took a bus the other way, into town. He got out in a busy street and threading down through the factory area he kept his bearings on the four huge smokestacks of the power station. Out of two of the smokestacks white plumes were rising calmly into the clear sky. When he got to the power station he was faced with an enormous high fence of iron staves with spiked tops and a tall steel gate, locked fast. He peered through the gate and saw some black men off duty, sitting in the sun on upturned boxes playing some kind of drafts game. He called them, and a big slow-moving man in brown overalls and a wide leather belt came over to talk.

André explained very carefully what he wanted. If they would switch off the current then he or somebody good at climbing could go up and save the swallow. The man smiled broadly and clicked his tongue. He shouted something at the others and they laughed. His

Words to Know

impudently (IM pyoo duhnt lee) *adv.*: Shamelessly; disrespectfully

menacing (MEN uhs ing) *adj.*: Threatening

name, he said, was Gas—Gas Makabeni. He was just a maintenance boy and he couldn't switch off the current. But he unlocked a steel frame-door in the gate and let André in.

"Ask them in there," he said, grinning. André liked Gas very much. He had ESCOM in big cloth letters on his back and he was friendly, opening the door like that. André went with Gas through a high arched entrance and at once he seemed to be surrounded with the vast awesome hum of the power station. It made him feel jumpy. Gas took him to a door and pushed him in. A white engineer in overalls questioned him and he smiled too.

"Well," he said. "Let's see what can be done."

He led him down a long corridor and up a short cut of steel zigzag steps. Another corridor came to an enormous paneled hall with banks of dials and glowing lights and men in long white coats sitting in raised chairs or moving about silently. André's heart was pounding good and fast. He could hear the humming sound strongly and it seemed to come from everywhere, not so much a sound as a feeling under his feet.

The engineer in overalls handed him over to one of the men at the control panels and he was so nervous by this time he took a long while trying to explain about the swallow. The man had to ask him a lot of questions and he got tongue-tied and could not give clear answers. The man did not smile at all. He went off and a minute later came and fetched André to a big office. A black-haired man with glasses was sitting at a desk. On both sides of the desk were telephones and panels of push-buttons. There was a carpet on the floor and huge leather easy chairs. The whole of one wall was a large and exciting circuit map with flickering colored lights showing where the power was going all over the country.

André did not say five words before his lip began trembling and two tears rolled out of his eyes. The man told him, "Sit down, son, and don't be scared."

Then the man tried to explain. How could they cut off the power when thousands and thousands of machines were running on electricity? He pointed with the back of his pencil at the circuit map. If there were a shutdown the power would have to be rerouted, and that meant calling in other power stations and putting a heavy load on the lines. Without current for one minute the trains would stop, hospitals would go dark in the middle of an operation, the mine skips would suddenly halt twelve thousand feet down. He knew André was worried about the swallow, only things like that just happened and that was life.

"Life?" André said, thinking it was more like death.

The big man smiled. He took down the boy's name and address, and he said, "You've done your best, André. I'm sorry I can't promise you anything."

Downstairs again, Gas Makabeni let him out at the gate. "Are they switching off the power?" Gas asked.

"No."

Mayi babo! Gas shook his head and clicked. But he did not smile this time. He could see the boy was very unhappy.

André got home hours late and his mother was frantic. He lied to her too, saying he had been detained after school. He kept his eyes away from the powerline and did not have the stomach to look for the swallow. He felt so bad about it because they were all letting it die. Except for the other swallows that brought it food it would be dead already.

And that was life, the man said. . . .

It must have been the middle of the night when he woke up. His mother was in the room and the light was on.

"There's a man come to see you," she said. "Did you ask anyone to come here?"

"No, Mama," he said, dazed.

"Get up and come." She sounded cross and he was scared stiff. He went out on to the stoop and there he saw his father in his pajamas and the back of a big man in brown overalls with ESCOM on them: a black man. It was Gas Makabeni!

"Gas!" he shouted. "Are they going to do it?"

"They're doing it," Gas said.

A linesman and a truck driver came up the steps on the stoep.[8] The lineman explained to André's father a maintenance switch-down had been ordered at minimum-load hour. He wanted to be shown where the bird was. André glanced, frightened, at his father who nodded and said, "Show him."

He went in the maintenance truck with the man and the driver and Gas. It took them only five minutes to get the truck in position under the power. The maintenance man checked the time and they began running up the extension ladder. Gas hooked a chain in his broad belt and pulled on his flashlight helmet. He swung out on the ladder and began running up it as if he had no weight at all. Up level with the pylon insulators, his flashlight picked out the swallow hanging on the dead wire. He leaned over and carefully worked the bird's tiny claw loose from the wire binding and then he put the swallow in the breast pocket of his overalls.

In a minute he was down again and he took the bird out and handed it to the boy. André could see even in the light of the flashlamp that the swallow had faint grey fringes round the edges of its shining blue-black feathers and that meant it was a young bird. This was its first year. He was almost speechless, holding the swallow in his hands and feeling its slight quiver.

"Thanks," he said. "Thanks, Gas. Thanks, sir."

His father took the swallow from him at the house and went off to find a box to keep it out of reach of the cats.

"Off you go to bed now," the mother said. "You've had quite enough excitement for one day."

The swallow drank thirstily but would not eat anything, so the parents thought it best to let it go as soon as it would fly. André took the box to his fort near the gum tree and looked towards the koppie and the powerline. It was early morning and dew sparkled on the overhead wires and made the whole level veld gleam like a magic inland sea. He held the swallow in his cupped hands and it lay there quiet with the tips of its wings crossed. Suddenly it took two little jumps with its tiny claws and spread its slender wings. Frantically they beat the air. The bird seemed to be dropping to the ground. Then it skimmed forward only a foot above the grass.

He remembered long afterwards how, when it really took wing and began to gain height, it gave a little shiver of happiness, as if it knew it was free.

---

8. stoep (STOOP) *n.*: A stoop; a small porch or platform with steps at the entrance of a house.

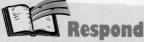

Respond

- Were you surprised by the power company's response to the boy's request? Why or why not?
- With a partner, role-play a discussion between André's parents the day that he frees the bird.

Activities

MAKE MEANING

Explore Your Reading

Look Back (Recall)

1. List the steps André takes to save the trapped swallow.

Think It Over (Interpret)

2. Why do you think André is lonely?
3. How does he feel about the power line and the swallows?
4. Why does he care so much about the trapped bird?
5. How is the title of the story a clue to the way that André changes?

Go Beyond (Apply)

6. How does this story answer the question "What is my responsibility to others?"

Develop Reading and Literary Skills

Analyze Symbols

Your chart has shown you how the author uses the swallows and the power line as **symbols** that stand for more than themselves. André is a "lonely" boy who likes to fill "the empty spaces in his life by imagining things." The power line takes "his thoughts away into a magical distance," and so do the birds. They symbolize his connection with a larger world.

1. What qualities of the power line and the birds make them good symbols of a link to the larger world?
2. What do you think the trapped bird symbolizes? Explain.
3. In what ways is André, like the swallow, trapped in his world?
4. How is his freeing of the swallow a symbol?

Ideas for Writing

André's courage and persistence inspire other characters to do what is right and affect a large company.

Monologue Write a speech in which Gas Makabeni tells his wife about the freeing of the swallow. Have him express his thoughts and feelings about the rescue, his part in it, and André's visit to the gas company.

Company Report Imagine that you are a manager at the power company. Write a report about the electrical shutdown, explaining the reasons for it and outlining the results. Use a memo format if you wish.

Ideas for Projects

Teens Who Made a Difference Like André, young people throughout history have tried to make a difference. Research events like the Children's Crusade and figures like Joan of Arc. Present your findings in the form of an annotated and illustrated time line. [Social Studies Link; Art Link]

Animal Rescue and Protection Acting in the same spirit as André does, groups like the Sierra Club and the Audubon Society have rescued birds from oil slicks, lobbied to save whales, and educated others about protecting animals. Research some of their activities, and present your findings to your classmates. [Science Link]

South African Background This story is set in South Africa. In a bulletin board display, explain how its leaders, white and black, thought about their responsibilities to others. Ask your social studies teacher for help in researching your display. [Social Studies Link]

How Am I Doing?

Take a moment to answer these questions:
What have I learned about symbols? How can I apply what I've learned about symbols to other stories?

What did I learn from this story about my responsibility to others?

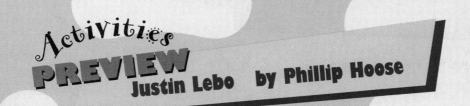

Activities
PREVIEW
Justin Lebo by Phillip Hoose

How can I help others by doing what I enjoy?

Reach Into Your Background

Sometimes helping others and enjoying oneself seem like opposing ideas. However, if you think about it, enjoyment is not always selfish. You can probably remember a time when you felt better just because you helped someone. Also, the things you really love to do may help others more than you imagine.

Continue thinking about this by doing one or both of these activities:

- Freewrite about a hobby, subject, or sport you love. Focus on ways in which your interest does or could help others.
- In a small group, tell about a time when helping others made you feel better about yourself.

Read Actively
Make Inferences About the Subject of a Biography

This story of Justin Lebo's life written by someone else, a **biography,** shows how he helped others *and* enjoyed himself. In reading any biography, you can **make inferences,** guesses based on evidence, about the subject. For example, if someone loves to fix bikes, you can infer that he or she has mechanical ability. By making inferences, you can learn more about the subject of a biography than the author tells you directly.

As you read "Justin Lebo," make inferences about him by filling in an inference map like this one.

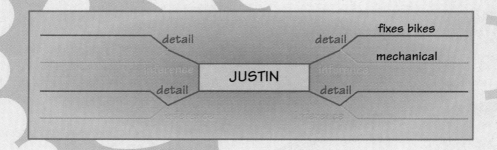

Justin Lebo

Phillip Hoose

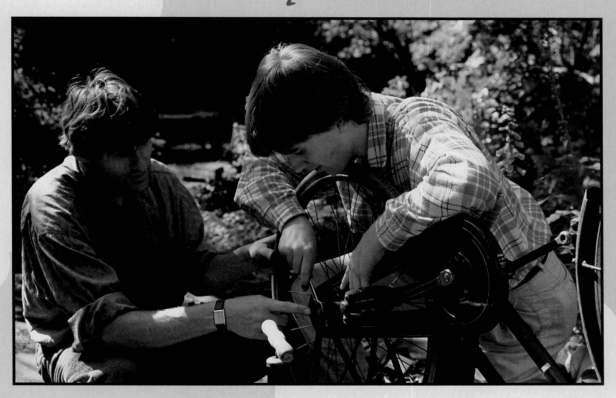

Something about the battered old bicycle at the garage sale caught ten-year-old Justin Lebo's eye. What a wreck! It was like looking at a few big bones in the dust and trying to figure out what kind of dinosaur they had once belonged to.

It was a BMX bike with a twenty-inch frame. Its original color was buried beneath five or six coats of gunky paint. Now it showed up as sort of a rusted red. Everything—the grips, the pedals, the brakes, the seat, the spokes—was bent or broken, twisted and rusted. Justin stood back as if he were inspecting a painting for sale at an auction. Then he made his final judgment: perfect.

Justin talked the owner down to $6.50 and asked his mother, Diane, to help him

Words to Know

battered (BAT uhrd) *adj*.: Damaged; worn out

load the bike into the back of their car.

When he got it home, he wheeled the junker into the garage and showed it proudly to his father. "Will you help me fix it up?" he asked. Justin's hobby was bike racing, a passion the two of them shared. Their garage barely had room for the car anymore. It was more like a bike shop. Tires and frames hung from hooks on the ceiling, and bike wrenches dangled from the walls.

After every race, Justin and his father would adjust the brakes and realign[1] the wheels of his two racing bikes. This was a lot of work, since Justin raced flat out, challenging every gear and part to perform to its fullest. He had learned to handle almost

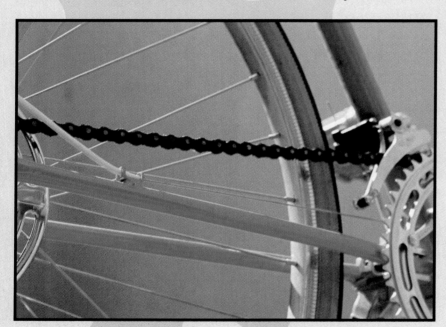

every repair his father could and maybe even a few things he couldn't. When Justin got really stuck, he went to see Mel, the owner of the best bike shop in town. Mel let him hang out and watch, and he even grunted a few syllables of advice from between the spokes of a wheel now and then.

---

1. **realign** (ree uh LĪN) *v.*: Readjust the parts so they work well together.

Now Justin and his father cleared out a work space in the garage and put the old junker up on a rack. They poured alcohol on the frame and rubbed until the old paint began to yield, layer by layer. They replaced the broken pedal, tightened down a new seat, and restored the grips. In about a week, it looked brand new.

Justin wheeled it out of the garage, leapt aboard, and started off around the block. He stood up and mashed down on the pedals, straining for speed. It was a good, steady ride, but not much of a thrill compared to his racers.

Soon he forgot about the bike. But the very next week, he bought another junker at a yard sale and fixed it up, too. After a while it bothered him that he wasn't really using either bike. Then he realized that what he loved about the old bikes wasn't riding them: it was the challenge of making something new and useful out of something old and broken.

Justin wondered what he should do with them. They were just taking up space in the garage. He remembered that when he was younger, he used to live near a large brick building called the Kilbarchan Home for Boys. It was a place for boys whose parents couldn't care for them for one reason or another.

He found "Kilbarchan" in the phone book and called the director, who said the boys would be thrilled to get two bicycles. The next day when Justin and his mother unloaded the bikes at the home, two boys raced out to greet them. They leapt aboard the bikes and started tooling around the semicircular driveway, doing wheelies and pirouettes, laughing and shouting.

The Lebos watched them for a while, then started to climb into their car to go home. The boys cried after them, "Wait a minute! You forgot your bikes!" Justin explained that the bikes were for them to keep. "They were so happy," Justin remembers. "It was like they couldn't believe it. It made me feel good to see them happy."

On the way home, Justin was silent. His mother assumed he was lost in a feeling of satisfaction. But he was thinking about what would happen once those bikes got wheeled inside and everyone saw them. How would all those kids decide who got the bikes? Two bikes could cause more trouble than they would solve. Actually, they hadn't been that hard to build. It was fun. Maybe he could do more. . . .

📖 **Read Actively**

Make an inference about Justin's character. What kind of person do his thoughts show he is?

"Mom," Justin said as they turned onto their street, "I've got an idea. I'm going to make a bike for every boy at Kilbarchan for Christmas." Diane Lebo looked at Justin out of the corner of her eye. She had rarely seen him so determined.

When they got home, Justin called Kilbarchan to find out how many boys lived there. There were twenty-one. It was already June. He had six months to make nineteen

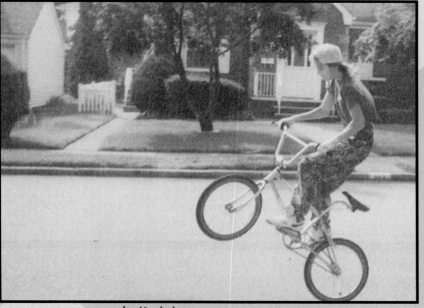

Justin Lebo

bikes. That was almost a bike a week. Justin called the home back to tell them of his plan. "I could tell they didn't think I could do it," Justin remembers. "I knew I could."

Justin knew his best chance was to build bikes almost the way GM or Ford builds cars: in an assembly line. He would start with frames from three-speed, twenty-four-inch BMX bicycles. They were common bikes, and all the parts were interchangeable. If he could find enough decent frames, he could take parts off broken bikes and fasten them onto the good frames. He figured it would take three or four junkers to produce enough parts to make one good bike. That meant sixty to eighty bikes. Where would he get them?

Garage sales seemed to be the only hope. It was June, and there would be garage sales all summer long. But even if he could find that many bikes, how could he ever pay for them? That was hundreds of dollars.

He went to his parents with a proposal. "When Justin was younger, say five or six,"

Words to Know

yield (YEELD) *v.*: Give way to pressure or force

says his mother, "he used to give some of his allowance away to help others in need. His father and I would donate a dollar for every dollar Justin donated. So he asked us if it could be like the old days, if we'd match every dollar he put into buying old bikes. We said yes."

Justin and his mother spent most of June and July hunting for cheap bikes at garage sales and thrift shops. They would haul the bikes home, and Justin would start stripping them down in the yard.

But by the beginning of August, he had managed to make only ten bikes. Summer vacation was

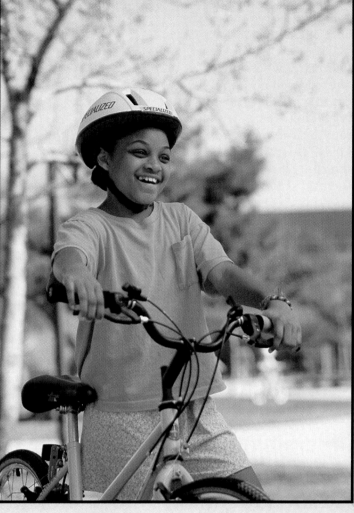

📖 **Read Actively**

Predict whether Justin will reach his goal.

almost over, and school and home-work would soon cut into his time. Garage sales would dry up when it got colder, and Justin was out of money. Still, he was deter-mined to find a way.

At the end of August, Justin got a break. A neighbor wrote a letter to the local newspaper de-scribing Justin's project, and an editor thought it would make a good story. One day a reporter entered the Lebo garage. Stepping gingerly through the tires and frames that covered the floor, she found a boy with cut fingers and dirty nails, banging a seat onto a frame. His clothes were covered with grease. In her admiring article about a boy who was devoting his summer to help kids he didn't even know, she said Justin needed bikes and money, and she printed his home phone number.

Overnight, everything changed. "There must have been a hundred calls," Justin says. "People would call me up and ask me to come over and pick up their old bike. Or

I'd be working in the garage, and a station wagon would pull up. The driver would leave a couple of bikes by the curb. It just snowballed."

By the start of school, the garage was overflowing with BMX frames. Pyramids of pedals and seats rose in the corners. Soon bike parts filled a toolshed in the backyard and then spilled out into the small yard itself, wearing away the lawn.

More and more writers and television and radio reporters called for interviews. Each time he told his story, Justin asked for bikes and money. "The first few interviews were fun," Justin says, "but it reached a point where I really didn't like doing them. The publicity was necessary, though. I had to keep doing interviews to get the donations I needed."

By the time school opened, he was working on ten bikes at a time. There were so many calls now that he was beginning to refuse offers that weren't the exact bikes he needed.

As checks came pouring in, Justin's money problems disappeared. He set up a bank account and began to make bulk orders of common parts from Mel's bike shop. Mel seemed delighted to see him. Sometimes, if Justin brought a bike by the shop, Mel would help him fix it. When Justin tried to talk him into a lower price for big orders, Mel smiled and gave in. He respected another good businessman. They became friends.

The week before Christmas Justin delivered the last of the twenty-one bikes to Kilbarchan. Once again, the boys poured out of the home and leapt aboard the bikes, tearing around the snow.

And once again, their joy inspired Justin. They reminded him how important bikes were to him. Wheels meant freedom. He thought how much more the freedom to ride must mean to boys like these who had so little freedom in their lives. He decided to keep on building.

"First I made eleven bikes for the children in a foster home my mother told me about. Then I made bikes for all the women in a battered women's shelter. Then I made ten little bikes and tricycles for the kids in a home for children with AIDS. Then I made twenty-three bikes for the Paterson Housing Coalition."

In the four years since he started, Justin Lebo has made between 150 and 200 bikes and given them all away. He has been careful to leave time for his homework, his friends, his coin collection, his new interest in marine biology, and of course his own bikes.

Reporters and interviewers have asked Justin Lebo the same question over and over: "Why do you do it?" The question seems to make him uncomfortable. It's as if they want him to say what a great person he is. Their stories always make him seem like a saint, which he knows he isn't. "Sure it's nice of me to make the bikes," he says, "because I don't have to. But I want to. In part, I do it for myself. I don't think you can ever really do anything to help anybody else if it doesn't make you happy.

"Once I overheard a kid who got one of my bikes say, 'A bike is like a book; it opens up a whole new world.' That's how I feel, too. It made me happy to know that kid felt that way. That's why I do it."

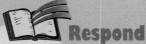

Respond

- Would you like to have someone like Justin Lebo as a friend? Why?
- What skills do you have to share? In a group, list some skills you have that could help others.

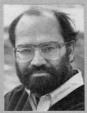

Phillip Hoose

Q: Why did Phillip Hoose write about Justin Lebo?
A: He wanted to include him in a book called *It's Our World, Too*. This book is about young people ages eight to seventeen who have worked to improve their world.
Q: What inspired the book?
A: Hoose wrote the book as a guide for young people who want to make a difference.

MAKE MEANING

Explore Your Reading

Look Back (Recall)

1. How does Justin accomplish his plan to help the boys at Kilbarchan?

Think It Over (Interpret)

2. Find two examples other than his plan for Kilbarchan that show Justin likes a challenge. Explain your choices.
3. In accomplishing his plan, how does Justin give inspiration to others and receive it from them?
4. What do you think is the most important thing Justin learns from his project? Explain.

Go Beyond (Apply)

5. What did you learn from this biography that you could apply to your life?

Develop Reading and Literary Skills

Evaluate a Biography

As you filled in your inference map, you learned what makes Justin Lebo special. Those who write **biographies,** accounts of someone else's life, look for subjects who stand out for one reason or another.

You can **evaluate,** or judge, a biography by seeing whether it meets certain standards. Excellent biographies will have the following elements:

- a subject who has achieved something important
- information that answers your questions about the subject
- dialogue, descriptions, and incidents that bring the subject to life

Use your inference map and other information from the story to answer these questions:

1. Find an example of each of these biographical elements in "Justin Lebo."
2. Evaluate this biography basing your answer on its use of the elements.

Ideas for Writing

Biographies tell the true stories of what real people have achieved. Folk tales often exaggerate the accomplishments of legendary characters.

Biographical Sketch Think about someone you know who has done something to make a difference. Then write a biographical sketch of that person. Make the person come alive by giving clues to his or her character.

Folk Tale Turn the biography of Justin Lebo into a folk tale by exaggerating his accomplishments. Make him into a larger-than-life character.

Ideas for Projects

Community Participation Justin Lebo worked by himself, but you may want to join an organization that helps others. Ask your guidance counselor for help in researching such an organization, and find out how you can work there as a volunteer. As you work, keep a journal to record your experiences. [Social Studies Link]

Proposal Chart Like Justin Lebo, think of ideas that could help your community—for example, a day-care center or new equipment in a local park. Make a chart to show how many people would be affected and how much money and time are necessary to make an improvement. To get started, check with your local government and the library. [Math Link]

How-to Fair Justin Lebo helped his community through his skill at fixing bikes. Organize a fair in which students demonstrate helpful skills to other students and members of the community.

How Am I Doing?

Respond to these questions in your journal:
What did I learn about making inferences? How will making inferences help me with my work in social studies, mathematics, and science?

How can I demonstrate what I learned about my responsibility to others?

What Is My Responsibility to Others?

Think Critically About the Selections

The selections in this section focus on the question "What is my responsibility to others?" On your own or with a partner, complete one or two of the following activities to show what you've learned. You can write your responses in a journal or share them in discussion.

1. Imagine you were writing a book about people who made a difference in the lives of others. Choose a character from this section, real or imaginary, to include in your book. Then tell how this character made a difference in someone else's life. **(Apply; Analyze)**

2. Choose a selection from this section that was especially meaningful for you. Use the theme of this selection as the inspiration for an original poem about responsibility to others. **(Synthesize)**

3. The selections you have read offer different answers to the question "What is my responsibility to others?" Choose two selections and compare and contrast what they say about our duty to others. **(Compare and Contrast)**

4. Choose individuals from several selections to participate in a panel discussion on "What is my responsibility to others?" Write a dialogue that expresses what these characters might say to one another as they tried to answer the question. **(Hypothesize)**

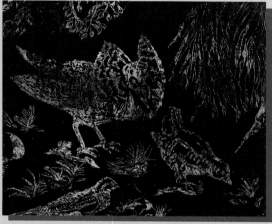

Student Art **Three Birds** Judit Santak Hungary, Paintbrush Diplomacy

Projects

Environmental Issues Project Through a local environmental organization, get involved in a stream or beach cleanup, a recycling program, or another project to improve the environment. Give an oral presentation to the class on the goals and achievements of your project. Perhaps others will volunteer to help you. [Science Link]

Responsibility Survey Interview people from many different walks of life and have them answer the question "What is my responsibility to others?" Record their answers, tally them, and then show which responsibilities scored highest because they were mentioned by the most people. [Math Link]

Mobile Create a mobile that represents our responsibilities to others. Include illustrations, photographs, and quotations to help communicate your ideas. Let each item on the mobile symbolize one responsibility. Write a key that explains your symbols. Hang your completed mobile in your classroom or make a display for the school library. [Art Link]

Looking at Forms:

Paul Zindel

Terms to know

A **drama** is a story written to be performed by actors.

The **plot,** or sequence of events in a drama, is based on a conflict, or problem, that characters must solve.

The **script,** or written form of a drama, includes both dialogue and stage directions.

Dialogue is the conversation that takes place among characters in a drama.

The **stage directions,** usually printed in italics, tell what the scene looks like and how actors should move and speak.

A restless ghost! What an exciting, grabbing image with which to start a play or any other story! It worked for the movie "Ghostbusters." It worked for William Shakespeare when he wrote *Hamlet*. In fact, Shakespeare often begins his plays with shocking images to get our attention.

A Christmas Carol: Scrooge and Marley, too, tells a story that starts with an explosive vision as startling as a mind-boggling rock video. For openers, we're asked to conjure up a collection of chicken sellers, weirdos, and ghastly spirits as shocking as any scary story could muster. More importantly, the images, dialogue, and action lead us to some really cool insights concerning human nature. Our challenge when reading a play is always to visualize—to see the story in the private movie theaters that are our minds.

A Cold, Dark Night First the playwright invites the computers of our brains to summon a vision of London on a Christmas Eve in 1843. It is a day when a grisly ghost has walked into Ebenezer Scrooge's miserly life and told him he'd better get his act together—or else! We call forth the image and chill of falling snow and creeping fog. We hear ghostly bells and music, crackle-voiced characters with frightening red eyes and shivering blue lips. We watch these characters *squeeze* and *grasp* and *shudder* on a night when specters walk. These are stirring "action" words from the playwright, and we know something truly horrible is going to happen. How delicious!

As we visualize, it's helpful to remember that most plays can be read as mystery stories. There are questions that grab onto our minds and hold tight. These questions usually center on the main characters as we begin to know them through the stage directions and dialogue. We try to see who the characters are, to glimpse what they're after, and what thrilling actions they're willing to take to reach their goals.

Literary Drama

Getting Involved in the Play The most important issue that haunts us is the key to a play's plot, or sequence of events. An important question to ask ourselves when reading a play is, "What's different about today than any other day?" The answer helps us to define the plot and to focus on our lead character's chief problem very quickly. In the best of plays, the main character's problem becomes our problem. It is then that we are hooked. *We must know what happens! We must know how it will all turn out! We must read on!*

Many young adults know **Paul Zindel's** (1936–) novels of growing up. With titles like *The Pigman* and *My Darling, My Hamburger,* Zindel captures readers' attention before they even begin. Once they start, readers find that they can't stop.

Zindel's Pulitzer Prize–winning play also has an interest-grabbing title: *The Effect of Gamma Rays on Man-in-the-Moon Marigolds.*

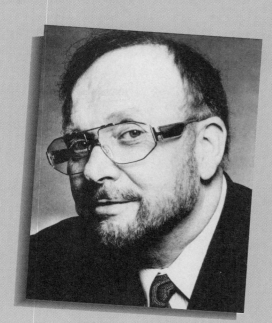

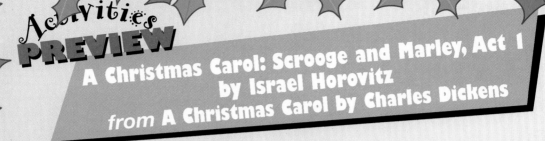

What can a live play offer that a movie can't?

Reach Into Your Background

Drama is everywhere—in movies, on television, and in plays. Your friends may talk about the latest movie or predict the ending of a miniseries. Drama clubs perform plays for classmates and relatives.

However, all dramatic presentations are not alike. Think about how watching a play is different from seeing a movie. Compare live drama to movies by doing one or both of these activities in a small group:

- Brainstorm to list similarities and differences between live drama and movies.
- Tell about roles you have had in school or community plays. Then reenact those roles for group members.

Read Actively
Identify Conflicts in Drama

Whether performed live or captured in film, a **drama** is a sequence of events based on conflicts, or struggles, between opposing sides. Unlike **conflicts** in stories, those in dramas are revealed only through **dialogue,** conversations between characters. When you read a drama, you can identify conflicts by looking for clues in the dialogue, like angry words. By identifying conflicts, you will understand what keeps the events in a drama moving.

As you read this play, pretend you are an audience of one sitting in a theater. Identify the conflicts of the main character, Scrooge, by listening to what he says and picturing what he does. In a chart like this one, note the conflicts you "hear" and "see."

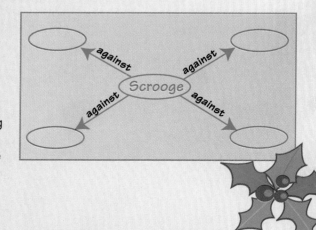

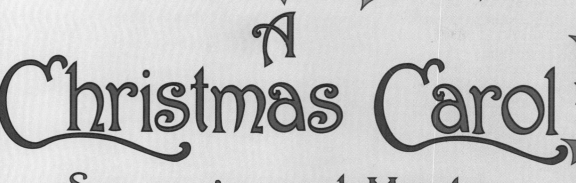

A Christmas Carol

Scrooge and Marley

Israel Horovitz
from A Christmas Carol
by Charles Dickens
Act I

THE PEOPLE OF THE PLAY

Jacob Marley, a specter

Ebenezer Scrooge, not yet dead, which is to say still alive

Bob Cratchit, Scrooge's clerk

Fred, Scrooge's nephew

Thin Do-Gooder

Portly Do-Gooder

Specters (Various), carrying moneyboxes

The Ghost of Christmas Past

Four Jocund Travelers

A Band of Singers

A Band of Dancers

Little Boy Scrooge

Young Man Scrooge

Fan, Scrooge's little sister

The Schoolmaster

Schoolmates

Fezziwig, a fine and fair employer

Dick, young Scrooge's co-worker

Young Scrooge

A Fiddler

More Dancers

Scrooge's Lost Love

Scrooge's Lost Love's Daughter

Scrooge's Lost Love's Husband

The Ghost of Christmas Present

Some Bakers

Mrs. Cratchit, Bob Cratchit's wife

Belinda Cratchit, a daughter

Martha Cratchit, another daughter

Peter Cratchit, a son

Tiny Tim Cratchit, another son

Scrooge's Niece, Fred's wife

The Ghost of Christmas Future, a mute Phantom

Three Men of Business

Drunks, Scoundrels, Women of the Streets

A Charwoman

Mrs. Dilber

Joe, an old second-hand goods dealer

A Corpse, very like Scrooge

An Indebted Family

Adam, a young boy

A Poulterer

A Gentlewoman

Some More Men of Business

THE PLACE OF THE PLAY

Various locations in and around the City of London, including Scrooge's Chambers and Offices; the Cratchit Home; Fred's Home; Scrooge's School; Fezziwig's Offices; Old Joe's Hide-a-Way.

THE TIME OF THE PLAY

The entire action of the play takes place on Christmas Eve, Christmas Day, and the morning after Christmas, 1843.

ACT I

Scene 1

[*Ghostly music in auditorium. A single spotlight on* JACOB MARLEY, *D.C. He is ancient; awful, dead-eyed. He speaks straight out to auditorium.*]

MARLEY. [*Cackle-voiced*] My name is Jacob Marley and I am dead. [*He laughs.*] Oh, no, there's no doubt that I am dead. The register of my burial was signed by the clergyman, the clerk, the undertaker . . . and by my chief mourner . . . Ebenezer Scrooge . . . [*Pause; remembers*] I am dead as a doornail.

[*A spotlight fades up, Stage Right, on* SCROOGE, *in his counting-house,*[1] *counting. Lettering on the window behind* SCROOGE *reads: "SCROOGE AND MARLEY, LTD." The spotlight is tight on* SCROOGE's *head*

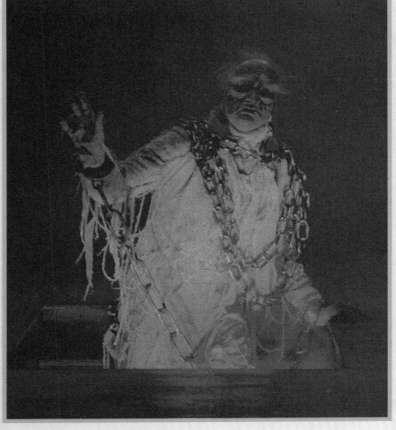

and shoulders. We shall not yet see into the offices and setting. Ghostly music continues, under. MARLEY *looks across at* SCROOGE; *pitifully. After a moment's pause*]

I present him to you: Ebenezer Scrooge . . . England's most tightfisted hand at the grindstone, Scrooge! a squeezing, wrenching, grasping, scraping, clutching, covetous, old sinner! secret, and self-contained, and solitary as an oyster. The cold within him freezes his old features, nips his pointed nose, shrivels his cheek, stiffens his gait; makes his eyes red, his thin lips blue; and speaks out shrewdly in his grating voice. Look at him. Look at him . . .

[SCROOGE *counts and mumbles.*]

---

1. **counting-house:** An office for keeping financial records and writing business letters.

SCROOGE. They owe me money and I will collect. I will have them jailed, if I have to. They owe me money and I will collect what is due me.

[MARLEY *moves toward* SCROOGE; *two steps. The spotlight stays with him.*]

MARLEY. [*Disgusted*] He and I were partners for I don't know how many years. Scrooge was my sole executor, my sole administrator, my sole assign, my sole residuary legatee,[2] my sole friend and my sole mourner. But Scrooge was not so cut up by the sad event of my death, but that he was an excellent man of business on the very day of my funeral, and solemnized[3] it with an undoubted bargain. [*Pauses again in disgust*] He never painted out my name from the window. There it stands, on the window and above the warehouse door: Scrooge and Marley. Sometimes people new to our business call him Scrooge and sometimes they call him Marley. He answers to both names. It's all the same to him. And it's cheaper than painting in a new sign, isn't it? [*Pauses; moves closer to* SCROOGE] Nobody has ever stopped him in the street to say, with gladsome looks, "My dear Scrooge, how are you? When will you come to see me?" No beggars implored him to bestow a trifle, no children ever ask him what it is o'clock, no man or woman now, or ever in his life, not once, inquire the way to such and such a place. [MARLEY *stands next to* SCROOGE *now. They share, so it seems, a spotlight.*] But what does Scrooge care of any of this? It is the very thing he likes! To edge his way along the crowded paths of life, warning all human sympathy to keep its distance.

[*A ghostly bell rings in the distance.* MARLEY *moves away from* SCROOGE, *now, heading D. again. As he does, he "takes" the light:* SCROOGE *has disappeared into the black void beyond.* MARLEY *walks D.C., talking directly to the audience. Pauses*]

The bell tolls and I must take my leave. You must stay a while with Scrooge and watch him play out his scroogey life. It is now the story: the once-upon-a-time. Scrooge is busy in his counting-house. Where else? Christmas eve and Scrooge is busy in his counting-house. It is cold, bleak, biting weather outside: foggy withal: and, if you listen closely, you can hear the people in the court go wheezing up and down, beating their hands upon their breasts, and stamping their feet upon the pavement stones to warm them . . .

[*The clocks outside strike three.*]

Only three! and quite dark outside already: it has not been light all day this day.

[*This ghostly bell rings in the distance again.* MARLEY *looks about him. Music in.* MARLEY *flies away.*] (N.B. MARLEY'S *comings and goings should, from time to time, induce the explosion of the odd flash-pot.* I.H.)

Scene 2

[*Christmas music in, sung by a live chorus, full. At conclusion of song, sound faces under and into the distance. Lights*

---

2. My sole executor (ig ZEK yuh tuhr), **my sole administrator, my sole assign** (uh SIN), **my sole residuary legatee** (ri ZIJ yoo ehr ee LEG uh tee): All legal terms giving one person responsibility to carry out the wishes of another who has died.

3. solemnized: (SAHL uhm nīzd) *v.*: Honored or remembered.

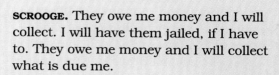

Words to Know

implored (im PLAWRD) *v.*: Asked or begged earnestly

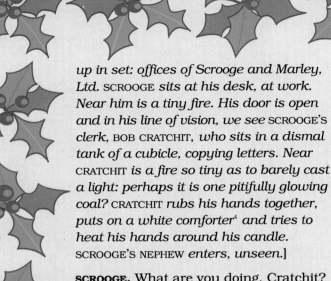

up in set: offices of Scrooge and Marley, Ltd. SCROOGE *sits at his desk, at work. Near him is a tiny fire. His door is open and in his line of vision, we see* SCROOGE'S *clerk,* BOB CRATCHIT, *who sits in a dismal tank of a cubicle, copying letters. Near* CRATCHIT *is a fire so tiny as to barely cast a light: perhaps it is one pitifully glowing coal?* CRATCHIT *rubs his hands together, puts on a white comforter⁴ and tries to heat his hands around his candle.* SCROOGE'S NEPHEW *enters, unseen.*]

SCROOGE. What are you doing, Cratchit? Acting cold, are you? Next, you'll be asking to replenish your coal from my coalbox, won't you? Well, save your breath, Cratchit! Unless you're prepared to find employ elsewhere!

NEPHEW. [*Cheerfully; surprising* SCROOGE] A merry Christmas to you, Uncle! God save you!

SCROOGE. Bah! Humbug!⁵

NEPHEW. Christmas a "humbug," Uncle? I'm sure you don't mean that.

SCROOGE. I do! Merry Christmas? What right do you have to be merry? What reason have you to be merry? You're poor enough!

NEPHEW. Come, then. What right have you to be dismal? What reason have you to be morose? You're rich enough.

SCROOGE. Bah! Humbug!

NEPHEW. Don't be cross, Uncle.

SCROOGE. What else can I be? Eh? When I live in a world of fools such as this? Merry Christmas? What's Christmas-time to you but a time of paying bills without any money; a time for finding yourself a year older, but not an hour richer. If I could work my will, every idiot who goes about with "Merry Christmas" on his lips, should be boiled with his own pudding, and buried with a stake of holly through his heart. He should!

NEPHEW. Uncle!

SCROOGE. Nephew! You keep Christmas in your own way and let me keep it in mine.

NEPHEW. Keep it! But you don't keep it, Uncle.

SCROOGE. Let me leave it alone, then. Much good it has ever done you!

NEPHEW. There are many things from which I have derived good, by which I have not profited, I daresay. Christmas among the rest. But I am sure that I always thought of Christmas time, when it has come round—as a good time: the only time I know of, when men and women seem to open their shut-up hearts freely, and to think of people below them as if they really were fellow-passengers to the grave, and not another race of creatures bound on other journeys. And therefore, Uncle, though it has never put a scrap of gold or silver in my pocket, I believe that it *has* done me good, and that it *will* do me good; and I say, God bless it!

[*The* CLERK *in the tank applauds, looks at the furious* SCROOGE *and pokes out his tiny fire, as if in exchange for the moment of impropriety.* SCROOGE *yells at him.*]

---

4. **comforter** (KUM fuhr tuhr) *n.:* A long woolen scarf.
5. **Humbug!** (HUM bug) *interj.:* Nonsense!

Words to Know

morose (muh ROHS) *adj.*: Gloomy; ill tempered

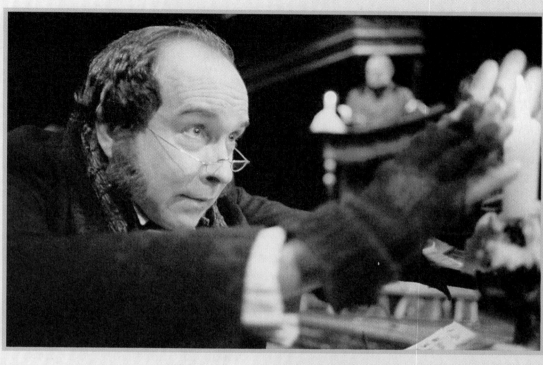

SCROOGE. [*To the* CLERK] Let me hear another sound from *you* and you'll keep your Christmas by losing your situation. [*To the* NEPHEW] You're quite a powerful speaker, sir. I wonder you don't go into Parliament.⁶

NEPHEW. Don't be angry, Uncle, Come! Dine with us tomorrow.

SCROOGE. I'd rather see myself dead than see myself with your family!

NEPHEW. But, why? Why?

SCROOGE. Why did you get married?

NEPHEW. Because I fell in love.

SCROOGE. That, sir, is the only thing that you have said to me in your entire life-time which is even more ridiculous than "Merry Christmas"! [*Turns from* NEPHEW] Good afternoon.

6. **Parliament** (PAHR luh muhnt): The national legislative body of Great Britain, in some ways like the United States Congress.

NEPHEW. Nay, Uncle, you never came to see me before I married either. Why give it as a reason for not coming now?

SCROOGE. Good afternoon, Nephew!

NEPHEW. I want nothing from you; I ask nothing of you; why cannot we be friends?

SCROOGE. Good afternoon!

NEPHEW. I am sorry with all my heart, to find you so resolute. But I have made the trial in homage to Christmas, and I'll keep my Christmas humor to the last. So A Merry Christmas, Uncle!

SCROOGE. Good afternoon!

NEPHEW. And A Happy New Year!

SCROOGE. Good afternoon!

NEPHEW. [*He stands facing* SCROOGE.] Uncle, you are the most . . . [*Pauses*] No, I shan't. My Christmas humor is intact

. . . [*Pause*] God bless you, Uncle . . . [NEPHEW *turns and starts for the door; he stops at* CRATCHIT's *cage.*] Merry Christmas, Bob Cratchit . . .

CRATCHIT. Merry Christmas to you sir, and a very, very happy New Year . . .

SCROOGE. [*Calling across to them*] Oh, fine, a perfection, just fine . . . to see the perfect pair of you: husbands, with wives and children to support . . . my clerk there earning fifteen shillings a week . . . and the perfect pair of you, talking about a Merry Christmas! [*Pauses*] I'll retire to Bedlam![7]

NEPHEW. [*To* CRATCHIT] He's impossible!

CRATCHIT. Oh, mind him not, sir. He's getting on in years, and he's alone. He's noticed your visit. I'll wager your visit has warmed him.

NEPHEW. Him? Uncle Ebenezer Scrooge? *Warmed?* You are a better Christian than I am, sir.

CRATCHIT. [*Opening the door for* NEPHEW; *two* DO-GOODERS *will enter, as* NEPHEW *exits.*] Good day to you, sir, and God bless.

NEPHEW. God bless . . . [*One man who enters is portly, the other is thin. Both are pleasant.*]

CRATCHIT. Can I help you, gentlemen?

THIN MAN. [*Carrying papers and books; looks around* CRATCHIT *to* SCROOGE] Scrooge and Marley's, I believe. Have I the pleasure of addressing Mr. Scrooge, or Mr. Marley?

SCROOGE. Mr. Marley has been dead these seven years. He died seven years ago this very night.

---

7. **Bedlam** (BED luhm): A hospital in London for the mentally ill.

PORTLY MAN. We have no doubt his liberality is well represented by his surviving partner . . . [*Offers his calling card*]

SCROOGE. [*Handing back the card; unlooked at*] . . . Good afternoon.

THIN MAN. This will take but a moment, sir . . .

PORTLY MAN. At this festive season of the year, Mr. Scrooge, it is more than usually desirable that we should make some slight provision for the poor and destitute, who suffer greatly at the present time. Many thousands are in want of common necessities; hundreds of thousands are in want of common comforts, sir.

SCROOGE. Are there no prisons?

PORTLY MAN. Plenty of prisons.

SCROOGE. And aren't the Union workhouses still in operation?

THIN MAN. They are. Still. I wish that I could say that they are not.

SCROOGE. The Treadmill[8] and the Poor Law[9] are in full vigor, then?

THIN MAN. Both very busy, sir.

SCROOGE. Ohhh, I see. I was afraid, from what you said at first, that something had occurred to stop them from their useful course. [*Pauses*] I'm glad to hear it.

PORTLY MAN. Under the impression that they scarcely furnish Christian cheer of

---

8. **Treadmill** (TRED mil): A kind of mill wheel turned by the weight of persons treading steps arranged around it; this device was used to punish prisoners in jails.

9. **the Poor Law**: The original 17th century Poor Laws called for overseers of the poor in each parish to provide relief for the needy. The New Poor Law of 1834 made the workhouses in which the poor sometimes lived and worked extremely harsh and unattractive. They became a symbol of the misery of the poor.

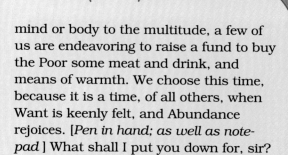

mind or body to the multitude, a few of us are endeavoring to raise a fund to buy the Poor some meat and drink, and means of warmth. We choose this time, because it is a time, of all others, when Want is keenly felt, and Abundance rejoices. [*Pen in hand; as well as note- pad*] What shall I put you down for, sir?

SCROOGE. Nothing!

PORTLY MAN. You wish to be left anony- mous?

SCROOGE. I wish to be left alone! [*Pauses; turns away; turns back to them*] Since you ask me what I wish, gentlemen, that is my answer. I help to support the establishments that I have mentioned: they cost enough: and those who are badly off must go there.

THIN MAN. Many can't go there; and many would rather die.

SCROOGE. If they would rather die, they had better do it, and decrease the sur- plus population. Besides—excuse me—I don't know that.

THIN MAN. But you might know it!

SCROOGE. It's not my business. It's enough for a man to understand his own business, and not to interfere with other people's. Mine occupies me constantly. Good afternoon, gentlemen! [SCROOGE *turns his back on the gentlemen and returns to his desk.*]

PORTLY MAN. But, sir, Mr. Scrooge . . . think of the poor.

SCROOGE. [*Turns suddenly to them. Pauses*] Take your leave of my offices, sirs, while I am still smiling.

[*The* THIN MAN *looks at the* PORTLY MAN. *They are undone. They*

shrug. *They move to door.* CRATCHIT *hops up to open it for them.*]

THIN MAN. Good day, sir . . . [*To* CRATCHIT] A Merry Christmas to you, sir . . .

CRATCHIT. Yes. A merry Christmas to both of you . . .

PORTLY MAN. Merry Christmas . . .

[CRATCHIT *silently squeezes something into the hand of the* THIN MAN.]

THIN MAN. What's this?

CRATCHIT. Shhhh . . .

[CRATCHIT *opens the door; wind and snow whistle into the room.*]

THIN MAN. Thank you, sir, thank you.

[CRATCHIT *closes the door and returns to his workplace.* SCROOGE *is at his own counting table. He talks to* CRATCHIT *with- out looking up.*]

SCROOGE. It's less of a time of year for being merry, and more a time of year for being loony . . . if you ask me.

CRATCHIT. Well, I don't know, sir . . .

[*The clock's bell strikes six o'clock.*]

Well, there it is, eh, six?

SCROOGE. Saved by six bells, are you?

CRATCHIT. I must be going home . . . [*He snuffs out his candle and puts on his hat.*] I hope you have a . . . very very lovely day tomorrow, sir . . .

SCROOGE. Hmmm. Oh, you'll be wanting the whole day tomorrow, I suppose?

Words to Know

destitute (DES tuh toot) *n.*: Living in complete poverty

CRATCHIT. If quite convenient, sir.

SCROOGE. It's not convenient, and it's not fair. If I was to stop half-a-crown for it, you'd think yourself ill-used, I'll be bound?

[CRATCHIT *smiles faintly.*]

CRATCHIT. I don't know, sir . . .

SCROOGE. And yet, you don't think me ill-used, when I pay a day's wages for no work . . .

CRATCHIT. It's only but once a year . . .

SCROOGE. A poor excuse for picking a man's pocket every 25th of December! But I suppose you must have the whole day. Be here all the earlier the next morning!

CRATCHIT. Oh, I will, sir. I will. I promise you. And, sir . . .

SCROOGE. Don't say it, Cratchit.

CRATCHIT. But let me wish you a . . .

SCROOGE. Don't say it, Cratchit. I warn you . . .

CRATCHIT. Sir!

SCROOGE. Cratchit!

[CRATCHIT *opens the door.*]

CRATCHIT. All right, then, sir . . . well . . . [*Suddenly*] Merry Christmas, Mr. Scrooge!

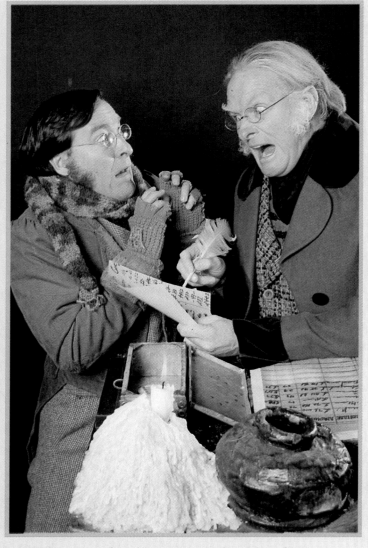

[*And he runs out the door, shutting same behind him.* SCROOGE *moves to his desk; gathering his coat, hat, etc. A* BOY *appears at his window. . . .*]

BOY. [*Singing*] "Away in a manger . . .".

[SCROOGE *seizes his ruler and whacks at the image of the* BOY *outside. The* BOY *leaves.*]

SCROOGE. Bah! Humbug! Christmas! Bah! Humbug! [*He shuts out the light.*]

A note on the crossover, following Scene 2: [SCROOGE *will walk alone to his rooms from his offices. As he makes a long slow cross of the stage, the scenery should change. Christmas music will be heard, various people will cross by* SCROOGE, *often smiling happily.*

There will be occasional pleasant greetings tossed at him.

SCROOGE, *in contrast to all, will grump and mumble. He will snap at passing boys, as might a horrid old hound.*

In short, SCROOGE'S *sounds and movements will define him in contrast from all other people who cross the stage: he is the* misanthrope, *the malcontent, the miser. He is* SCROOGE.

This statement of SCROOGE'S *character, by contrast to all other characters, should seem comical to the audience.*

During SCROOGE'S *crossover to his rooms, snow should begin to fall. All passers-by will hold their faces to the sky, smiling, allowing snow to shower them lightly.* SCROOGE, *by contrast, will bat at the flakes with his walking-stick, as might an insomniac swat at a sleep-stopping, middle-of-the-night swarm of mosquitoes. He will comment on the blackness of the night, and, finally, reach his rooms and his encounter with the magical specter:*[10] MARLEY, *his eternal mate.*]

---

10. specter (SPEK tur) *n.*: Ghost.

Scene 3

SCROOGE. No light at all . . . no moon . . . *that* is what is at the center of a Christmas Eve: dead black: void . . .

[SCROOGE *puts his key in the door's key-hole. He has reached his rooms now. The door knocker changes and is now* MAR-LEY'S *face. A musical sound; quickly: ghostly.* MARLEY'S *image is not at all angry, but looks at* SCROOGE *as did the old* MARLEY *look at* SCROOGE. *The hair is curiously stirred; eyes wide open, dead: absent of focus.* SCROOGE *stares wordlessly here. The face, before his very eyes, does deliquesce.*[11] *It is a knocker again.* SCROOGE *opens the door and checks the back of same, probably for* MARLEY'S *pigtail. Seeing nothing but screws and nuts,* SCROOGE *refuses the memory.*]

Pooh, pooh!

[*The sound of the door closing resounds throughout the house as thunder. Every room echoes the sound.* SCROOGE *fastens the door and walks across the hall to the stairs, trimming his candle as he goes; and then he goes slowly up the staircase. He checks each room: sitting room, bedroom, lumber-room. He looks under the sofa, under the table: nobody there. He fixes his evening gruel on the hob,*[12] *changes his jacket.* SCROOGE *sits near the tiny low-flamed fire, sipping his gruel. There are various pictures on the walls: all of them now show likenesses of* MAR-LEY. SCROOGE *blinks his eyes.*]

Bah! Humbug!

[SCROOGE *walks in a circle about the room. The pictures change back into their*

---

11. deliquesce (del uh KWES) *v.*: Melt away.
12. gruel (GROO uhl) **on the hob** (HAHB): A thin broth warming on a ledge at the back or side of the fireplace.

natural images. He sits down at the table in front of the fire. A bell hangs overhead. It begins to ring, of its own accord. Slowly, surely, begins the ringing of every bell in the house. They continue ringing for nearly half a minute. SCROOGE *is stunned by the phenomenon. The bells cease their ringing all at once. Deep below* SCROOGE, *in the basement of the house, there is a sound of clanking, of some enormous chain being dragged across the floors; and now up the stairs. We hear doors flying open.*]

Bah still! Humbug still! This is not happening! I won't believe it!

[MARLEY'S *ghost enters the room. He is horrible to look at: pigtail, vest, suit as usual, but he drags an enormous chain now, to which is fastened cash-boxes, keys, padlocks, ledgers, deeds, and heavy purses fashioned of steel. He is transparent.* MARLEY *stands opposite the stricken* SCROOGE.]

How now! What do you want of me?

MARLEY. Much!

SCROOGE. Who are you?

MARLEY. Ask me who I *was.*

SCROOGE. Who *were* you then?

MARLEY. In life, I was your business partner: Jacob Marley.

SCROOGE. I see . . . can you sit down?

MARLEY. I can.

SCROOGE. Do it then.

MARLEY. I shall. [MARLEY *sits opposite* SCROOGE, *in the chair across the table, at the front of the fireplace.*] You don't believe in me.

SCROOGE. I don't.

MARLEY. Why do you doubt your senses?

SCROOGE. Because every little thing affects them. A slight disorder of the stomach makes them cheat. You may be an undigested bit of beef, a blot of mustard, a crumb of cheese, a fragment of an underdone potato. There's more of gravy than of grave about you, whatever you are!

[*There is a silence between them.* SCROOGE *is made nervous by it. He picks up a toothpick.*]

Humbug! I tell you: humbug!

[MARLEY *opens his mouth and screams a ghostly, fearful scream. The scream echoes about each room of the house. Bats fly, cats screech, lightning flashes.* SCROOGE *stands and walks backwards against the wall.* MARLEY *stands and screams again. This time, he takes his head and lifts it from his shoulders. His head continues to scream.* MARLEY'S *face again appears on every picture in the room: all screaming.* SCROOGE, *on his knees before* MARLEY]

Mercy! Dreadful apparition,[13] mercy! Why, O! why do you trouble me so?

MARLEY. Man of the worldly mind, do you believe in me, or not?

SCROOGE. I do. I must. But why do spirits such as you walk the earth? And why do they come to me?

MARLEY. It is required of every man that the spirit within him should walk abroad among his fellow-men, and travel far and wide; and if that spirit goes not forth in life, it is condemned to do so after death. [MARLEY *screams*

---

13. apparation (ap uh RISH uhn) *n.*: Ghost.

again; a tragic scream; from his ghostly bones.] I wear the chain I forged in life. I made it link by link, and yard by yard. Is its pattern strange to *you?* Or would you know, you, Scrooge, the weight and length of the strong coil you bear yourself? It was full as heavy and long as this, seven Christmas Eves ago. You have labored on it, since. It is a ponderous chain.

[*Terrified that a chain will appear about his body,* SCROOGE *spins and waves the unwanted chain away. None, of course, appears. Sees* MARLEY *watching him dance about the room.* MARLEY *watches* SCROOGE; *silently.*]

SCROOGE. Jacob. Old Jacob Marley, tell me more. Speak comfort to me, Jacob . . .

MARLEY. I have none to give. Comfort comes from other regions, Ebenezer Scrooge, and is conveyed by other ministers, to other kinds of men. A very little more, is all that is permitted to me. I cannot rest, I cannot stay, I cannot linger anywhere . . . [*He moans again.*] my spirit never walked beyond our counting-house—mark me!—in life my spirit never roved beyond the narrow limits of our money-changing hole; and weary journeys lie before me!

SCROOGE. But you were always a good man of business, Jacob.

MARLEY. [*Screams word "business"; a flashpot explodes with him.*] BUSI-NESS!!! Mankind was my business. The common welfare was my business; charity, mercy, forbearance, benevo-

lence, were, all, my business. [SCROOGE *is quaking.*] Hear me, Ebenezer Scrooge! My time is nearly gone.

SCROOGE. I will, but don't be hard upon me. And don't be flowery, Jacob! Pray!

MARLEY. How is it that I appear before you in a shape that you can see, I may not tell. I have sat invisible beside you many and many a day. That is no light part of my penance.[14] I am here tonight to warn you that you have yet a chance and hope of escaping my fate. A chance and hope of my procuring, Ebenezer.

SCROOGE. You were always a good friend to me. Thank'ee!

MARLEY. You will be haunted by Three Spirits.

SCROOGE. Would that be the chance and hope you mentioned, Jacob?

MARLEY. It is.

SCROOGE. I think I'd rather not.

MARLEY. Without their visits, you cannot hope to shun the path I tread. Expect the first one tomorrow, when the bell tolls one.

SCROOGE. Couldn't I take 'em all at once, and get it over, Jacob?

MARLEY. Expect the second on the next night at the same hour. The third upon the next night when the last stroke of twelve has ceased to vibrate. Look to see me no more. Others may, but you may not. And look that, for your own sake, you remember what has passed between us!

[MARLEY *places his head back upon his shoulders. He approaches the window*

Words to Know

ponderous (PAHN duhr uhs)
adj.: Very heavy; bulky

---

14. penance (PEN uhns) *n.*: Any suffering a person takes on to show sorrow for wrongdoing.

and beckons to SCROOGE *to watch. Outside the window, specters fly by, carrying money-boxes and chains. They make a confused sound of lamentation.* MARLEY, *after listening a moment, joins into their mournful dirge. He leans to the window and floats out into the bleak, dark night. He is gone.*]

SCROOGE. [*Rushing to the window*] Jacob! No, Jacob! Don't leave me! I'm frightened!

[*He sees that* MARLEY *has gone. He looks outside. He pulls the shutter closed, so that the scene is blocked from his view. All sound stops. After a pause, he re-opens the shutter and all is quiet, as it should be on Christmas Eve. Carolers carol out of doors, in the distance.* SCROOGE *closes the shutter and walks down the stairs. He examines the door by which* MARLEY *first entered.*]

No one here at all! Did I imagine all that? Humbug! [*He looks about the room.*] I did imagine it. It only happened in my foulest dream-mind, didn't it? An undigested bit of . . .

[*Thunder and lightning in the room; suddenly*]

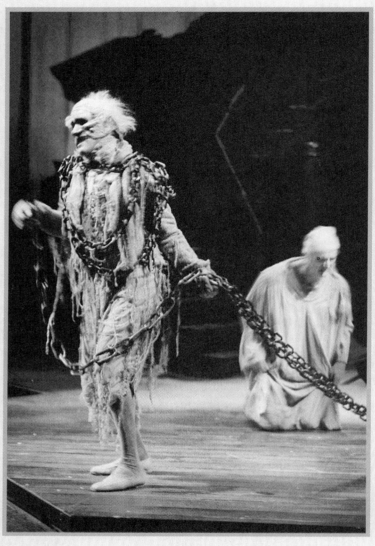

Sorry! Sorry!

[*There is silence again. The lights fade out.*]

Scene 4
[*Christmas music, choral, "Hark the Herald Angels Sing," sung by an onstage choir of children, spotlighted. D.C. Above,* SCROOGE *in his bed, dead to the world, asleep, in his darkened room. It should appear that the choir is singing somewhere outside of the house, of course,*

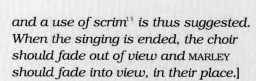

and a use of scrim[15] is thus suggested. When the singing is ended, the choir should fade out of view and MARLEY should fade into view, in their place.]

MARLEY. [*Directly to audience*] From this point forth . . . I shall be quite visible to you, but invisible to him. [*Smiles*] He will feel my presence, nevertheless, for, unless my senses fail me completely, we are—you and I—witness to the changing of a miser: that one, my partner in life, in business, and in eternity: that one: Scrooge. [*Moves to staircase, below* SCROOGE] See him now. He endeavors to pierce the darkness with his ferret eyes. [*To audience*] See him, now. He listens for the hour.

[*The bells toll.* SCROOGE *is awakened and quakes as the hour approaches one o'clock, but the bells stop their sound at the hour of twelve.*]

SCROOGE. [*Astonished*] Midnight! Why this isn't possible. It was past two when I went to bed. An icicle must have gotten into the clock's works! I couldn't have slept through the whole day and far into another night. It isn't possible that anything has happened to the sun, and this is twelve at noon! [*He runs to window; unshutters same; it is night.*] Night, still. Quiet, normal for the season, cold. It is certainly not noon. I cannot in any way afford to lose my days. Securities come due, promissory notes,[16] interest on investments: these are things that happen in the daylight! [*He returns to his bed.*] Was this a dream?

---

15. **scrim** (SKRIM) *n.*: A light, semitransparent curtain.

16. **promissory** (PRAHM i sawree) **notes:** Written promises to pay someone a certain amount of money.

[MARLEY *appears in his room. He speaks to the audience.*]

MARLEY. You see? He does not, with faith, believe in me fully, even still! Whatever will it take to turn the faith of a miser from money to men?

SCROOGE. Another quarter and it'll be one and Marley's ghosty friends will come. [*Pauses; listens*] Where's the chime for one? [*Ding, dong*] A quarter past [*Repeats*] Half-past! [*Repeats*] A quarter to it! But where's the heavy bell of the hour one? This is a game in which I lose my senses! Perhaps, if I allowed myself another short doze . . .

MARLEY. . . . Doze, Ebenezer, doze.

[*A heavy bell thuds its one ring; dull and definitely one o'clock. There is a flash of light.* SCROOGE *sits up, in a sudden. A hand draws back the curtains by his bed. He sees it.*]

SCROOGE. A hand! Who owns it! Hello!

[*Ghostly music again, but of a new nature to the play. A strange figure stands before* SCROOGE—*like a child, yet at the same time like an old man: white hair, but unwrinkled skin, long, muscular arms, but delicate legs and feet. Wears white tunic; lustrous belt cinches waist. Branch of fresh green holly in its hand, but has its dress trimmed with fresh summer flowers. Clear jets of light spring from the crown of its head. Holds cap in hand. The spirit is called PAST.*]

Are you the Spirit, sir, whose coming was foretold to me?

PAST. I am.

MARLEY. Does he take this to be a vision of his green grocer?

SCROOGE. Who, and what are you?

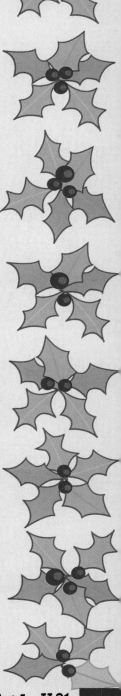

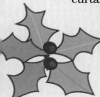

PAST. I am the Ghost of Christmas Past.

SCROOGE. Long past?

PAST. Your past.

SCROOGE. May I ask, please, sir, what business you have here with me?

PAST. Your welfare.

SCROOGE. Not to sound ungrateful, sir, and really, please do understand that I am plenty obliged for your concern, but, really, kind spirit, it would have done all the better for my welfare to have been left alone altogether, to have slept peacefully through this night.

PAST. Your reclamation, then. Take heed!

SCROOGE. My what?

PAST. [*Motioning to* SCROOGE *and taking his arm*] Rise! Fly with me! [*He leads* SCROOGE *to the window.*]

SCROOGE. [*Panicked*] Fly, but I am a mortal and cannot fly!

PAST. [*Pointing to his heart*] Bear but a touch of my hand *here* and you shall be upheld in more than this!

[SCROOGE *touches the* SPIRIT'S *heart and the lights dissolve into sparkly flickers. Lovely crystals of music are heard. The scene dissolves into another. Christmas music again*]

Scene 5

[SCROOGE *and the* GHOST OF CHRISTMAS PAST *walk together across an open stage. In the background, we see a field that is open; covered by a soft, downy snow: a country road.*]

SCROOGE. Good Heaven! I was bred in this place. I was a boy here!

[SCROOGE *freezes, staring at the field beyond.* MARLEY'S *ghost appears beside*

him; takes SCROOGE'S *face in his hands, and turns his face to the audience*]

MARLEY. You see this Scrooge: stricken by feeling. Conscious of a thousand odors floating in the air, each one connected with a thousand thoughts, and hopes, and joys, and care long, long forgotten. [*Pause*] This one—this Scrooge—before your very eyes, returns to life, among the living. [*To audience, sternly*] You'd best pay your most careful attention. I would suggest rapt.[17]

[*There is a small flash and puff of smoke and* MARLEY *is gone again.*]

PAST. Your lip is trembling, Mr. Scrooge. And what is that upon your cheek?

SCROOGE. Upon my cheek? Nothing . . . a blemish on the skin from the eating of overmuch grease . . . nothing . . . [*Suddenly*] Kind Spirit of Christmas Past, lead me where you will, but *quickly!* To be stagnant in this place is, for me, *unbearable!*

PAST. You recollect the way?

SCROOGE. Remember it! I would know it blindfolded! My bridge, my church, my winding river! [*Staggers about, trying to see it all at once. He weeps again.*]

PAST. These are but shadows of things that have been. They have no consciousness of us.

[*Four jocund travelers enter, singing a Christmas song in four-part harmony—* "God Rest Ye Merry, Gentlemen."]

SCROOGE. Listen! I know these men! I know them! I remember the beauty of their song!

---

17. rapt (RAPT) *adj.*: Giving complete attention; totally carried away by something.

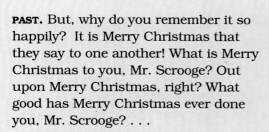

PAST. But, why do you remember it so happily? It is Merry Christmas that they say to one another! What is Merry Christmas to you, Mr. Scrooge? Out upon Merry Christmas, right? What good has Merry Christmas ever done you, Mr. Scrooge? . . .

SCROOGE. [*After a long pause*] None. No good. None . . . [*He bows his head.*]

PAST. Look, you, sir, a school ahead. The schoolroom is not quite deserted. A solitary child, neglected by his friends, is left there still.

[SCROOGE *falls to the ground; sobbing as he sees, and we see, a small boy, the young* SCROOGE, *sitting and weeping, bravely, alone at his desk: alone in a vast space, a void.*]

SCROOGE. I cannot look on him!

PAST. You must, Mr. Scrooge, you must.

SCROOGE. It's me. [*Pauses; weeps*] Poor boy. He lived inside his head . . . alone . . . [*Pauses; weeps*] poor boy. [*Pauses; stops his weeping*] I wish . . . [*Dries his eyes on his cuff*] ah! It's too late!

PAST. What is the matter?

SCROOGE. There was a boy singing a Christmas Carol outside my door last night. I should like to have given him something: that's all.

PAST. [*Smiles; waves his hand to* SCROOGE] Come. Let us see another Christmas.

[*Lights out on little boy. A flash of light. A puff of smoke. Lights up on older boy*]

SCROOGE. Look! Me, again! Older now! [*Realizes*] Oh, yes . . . still alone.

[*The boy—a slightly older* SCROOGE—*sits alone in a chair, reading. The door to* the room opens and a young girl enters. She is much, much younger than this slightly older SCROOGE. *She is, say, six, and he is, say, twelve. Elder* SCROOGE *and the* GHOST OF CHRISTMAS PAST *stand watching the scene, unseen.*]

FAN. Dear, dear brother, I have come to bring you home.

BOY. Home, little Fan?

FAN. Yes! Home, for good and all! Father is so much kinder than he ever used to be, and home's like heaven! He spoke so gently to me one dear night when I was going to bed that I was not afraid to ask him once more if you might come home; and he said "yes" . . . you should; and sent me in a coach to bring you. And you're to be a man and are never to come back here, but first, we're to be together all the Christmas long, and have the merriest time in the world.

BOY. You are quite a woman, little Fan!

[*Laughing; she drags at* BOY, *causing him to stumble to the door with her. Suddenly we hear a mean and terrible voice in the hallway. Off. It is the* SCHOOLMASTER.]

SCHOOLMASTER. Bring down Master Scrooge's travel box at once! He is to travel!

FAN. Who is that, Ebenezer?

BOY. O! Quiet, Fan. It is the Schoolmaster, himself!

[*The door bursts open and into the room bursts with it the* SCHOOLMASTER.]

SCHOOLMASTER. Master Scrooge?

BOY. Oh, Schoolmaster. I'd like you to meet my little sister, Fan, sir . . .

[*Two boys struggle on with* SCROOGE'S *trunk.*]

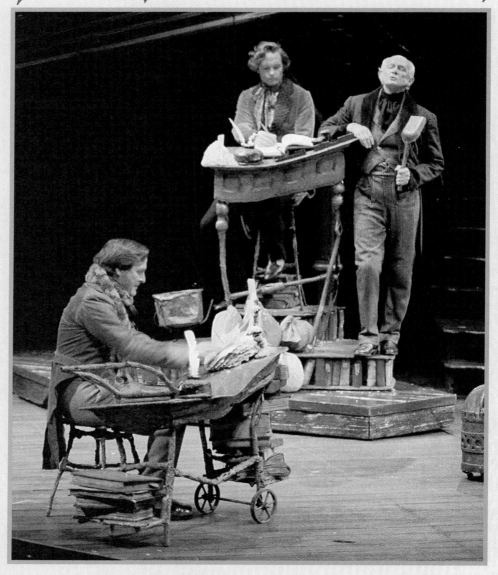

FAN. Pleased, sir . . . [*She curtsies.*]

SCHOOLMASTER. You are to travel, Master Scrooge.

SCROOGE. Yes, sir. I know sir . . .

[*All start to exit, but* FAN *grabs the coattail of the mean old* SCHOOLMASTER.]

BOY. Fan!

SCHOOLMASTER. What's this?

FAN. Pardon, sir, but I believe that you've forgotten to say your goodbye to my brother, Ebenezer, who stands still now awaiting it . . . [*She smiles, curtsies, lowers her eyes.*] pardon, sir.

SCHOOLMASTER. [*Amazed*] I . . . uh . . . harumph . . . uhh . . . well, then . . . [*Outstretches hand*] Goodbye, Scrooge.

BOY. Uh, well, goodbye, Schoolmaster . . .

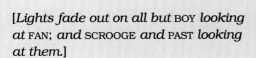

[*Lights fade out on all but* BOY *looking at* FAN; *and* SCROOGE *and* PAST *looking at them.*]

SCROOGE. Oh, my dear, dear little sister, Fan . . . how I loved her.

PAST. Always a delicate creature whom a breath might have withered, but she had a large heart . . .

SCROOGE. So she had.

PAST. She died a woman, and had, as I think, children.

SCROOGE. One child.

PAST. True. Your nephew.

SCROOGE. Yes.

PAST. Fine, then. We move on, Mr. Scrooge. That warehouse, there? Do you know it?

SCROOGE. Know it? Wasn't I apprenticed[18] there?

PAST. We'll have a look.

[*They enter the warehouse. The lights crossfade with them, coming up on an old man in Welsh wig:* FEZZIWIG.]

SCROOGE. Why, it's old Fezziwig! Bless his heart; it's Fezziwig, alive again!

[FEZZIWIG *sits behind a large, high desk, counting. He lays down his pen; looks at the clock; seven bells sound.*]

Quittin' time . . .

FEZZIWIG. Quittin' time . . . [*He takes off his waistcoat and laughs; calls off*] Yo ho, Ebenezer! Dick!

---

18. apprenticed (uh PREN tist) *v.*: Receiving financial support and instruction in a trade in return for work.

[DICK WILKINS *and* EBENEZER SCROOGE—*a young man version—enter the room.* DICK *and* EBENEZER *are* FEZZIWIG'S *apprentices.*]

SCROOGE. Dick Wilkins, to be sure! My fellow-'prentice! Bless my soul, yes. There he is. He was very much attached to me, was Dick. Poor Dick! Dear, dear!

FEZZIWIG. Yo ho, my boys. No more work tonight. Christmas Eve, Dick. Christmas, Ebenezer!

[*They stand at attention in front of* FEZZIWIG; *laughing.*]

Hilli-ho! Clear away, and let's have lots of room here! Hilli-ho, Dick! Chirrup, Ebenezer!

[*The young men clear the room, sweep the floor, straighten the pictures, trim the lamps, etc. The space is clear now. A fiddler enters, fiddling.*]

Hi-ho, Matthew! Fiddle away . . . where are my daughters?

[*The* FIDDLER *plays. Three young daughters of* FEZZIWIG *enter followed by six young male suitors. They are dancing to the music. All employees come in: workers, clerks, housemaids, cousins, the baker, etc. All dance. Full number wanted here. Throughout the dance, food is brought into the feast. It is "eaten" in dance, by the dancers.* EBENEZER *dances with all three of the daughters, as does* DICK. *They compete for the daughters, happily, in the dance.* FEZZIWIG *dances with his daughters.* FEZZIWIG *dances with* DICK *and* EBENEZER. *The music changes:* MRS. FEZZIWIG *enters. She lovingly scolds her husband. They dance. She dances with* EBENEZER, *lifting him and throwing him about. She is enormously fat. When the dance is ended, they all dance off, floating away, as does the music.*]

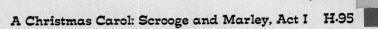

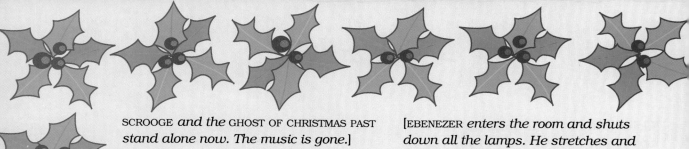

SCROOGE *and the* GHOST OF CHRISTMAS PAST *stand alone now. The music is gone.*]

PAST. It was a small matter, that Fezziwig made those silly folks so full of gratitude.

SCROOGE. Small!

PAST. Shhh!

[*Lights up on* DICK *and* EBENEZER]

DICK. We are blessed, Ebenezer, truly, to have such a master as Mr. Fezziwig!

YOUNG SCROOGE. He is the best, best, the very and absolute best! If ever I own a firm of my own, I shall treat my apprentices with the same dignity and the same grace. We have learned a wonderful lesson from the master, Dick!

DICK. Ah, that's a fact, Ebenezer. That's a fact!

PAST. Was it not a small matter, really? He spent but a few pounds[19] of his mortal money on your small party. Three or four pounds, perhaps. Is that so much that he deserves such praise as you and Dick so lavish now?

SCROOGE. It isn't that! It isn't that, Spirit. Fezziwig had the power to make us happy or unhappy; to make our service light or burdensome; a pleasure or a toil. The happiness he gave is quite as great as if it cost him a fortune.

PAST. What is the matter?

SCROOGE. Nothing particular.

PAST. Something, I think.

SCROOGE. No, no. I should like to be able to say a word or two to my clerk just now! That's all!

---

19. **pounds** (POWNDZ) *n.*: British currency.

[EBENEZER *enters the room and shuts down all the lamps. He stretches and yawns. The* GHOST OF CHRISTMAS PAST *turns to* SCROOGE; *all of a sudden.*]

PAST. My time grows short! Quick!

[*In a flash of light,* EBENEZER *is gone, and in his place stands an* OLDER SCROOGE, *this one a man in the prime of his life. Beside him stands a young woman in a mourning dress. She is crying. She speaks to the man, with hostility.*]

WOMAN. It matters little . . . to you, very little. Another idol has displaced me.

MAN. What idol has displaced you?

WOMAN. A golden one.

MAN. This is an even-handed dealing of the world. There is nothing on which it is so hard as poverty; and there is nothing it professes to condemn with such severity as the pursuit of wealth!

WOMAN. You fear the world too much. Have I not seen your nobler aspirations fall off one by one, until the master-passion, Gain, engrosses you? Have I not?

SCROOGE. No!

MAN. What then? Even if I have grown so much wiser, what then? Have I changed towards you?

WOMAN. No . . .

MAN. Am I?

WOMAN. Our contract is an old one. It was made when we were both poor and content to be so. You *are* changed. When it was made, you were another man.

MAN. I was not another man: I was a boy.

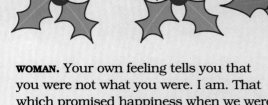

WOMAN. Your own feeling tells you that you were not what you were. I am. That which promised happiness when we were one in heart is fraught with misery now that we are two . . .

SCROOGE. No!

WOMAN. How often and how keenly I have thought of this, I will not say. It is enough that I *have* thought of it, and can release you . . .

SCROOGE. [*Quietly*] Don't release me, madame . . .

MAN. Have I ever sought release?

WOMAN. In words. No. Never.

MAN. In what then?

WOMAN. In a changed nature; in an altered spirit. In everything that made my love of any worth or value in your sight. If this has never been between us, tell me, would you seek me out and try to win me now? Ah, no!

SCROOGE. Ah, yes!

MAN. You think not?

WOMAN. I would gladly think otherwise if I could, heaven knows! But if you were free today, tomorrow, yesterday, can even I believe that you would choose a dowerless girl—you who in your very confidence with her weigh everything by Gain; or, choosing her, do I not know that your repentance and regret would surely follow? I do; and I release you. With a full heart, for the love of him you once were.

SCROOGE. Please, I . . . I . . .

MAN. Please, I . . . I . . .

WOMAN. Please. You may—the memory of what is past half makes me hope you will—

have pain in this. A very, very brief time, and you will dismiss the memory of it, as an unprofitable dream, from which it happened well that you awoke. May you be happy in the life that you have chosen for yourself . . .

SCROOGE. No!

WOMAN. Yourself . . . alone . . .

SCROOGE. No!

WOMAN. Goodbye, Ebenezer . . .

SCROOGE. Don't let her go!

MAN. Goodbye.

SCROOGE. No!

[*She exits.* SCROOGE *goes to younger man: himself.*]

You fool! Mindless loon! You fool!

MAN. [*To exited woman*] Fool. Mindless loon. Fool . . .

SCROOGE. Don't say that! Spirit, remove me from this place.

PAST. I have told you these were shadows of the things that have been. They are what they are. Do not blame me, Mr. Scrooge.

SCROOGE. Remove me! I cannot bear it!

[*The faces of all who appeared in this scene are now projected for a moment around the stage: enormous, flimsy, silent.*]

Leave me! Take me back! Haunt me no longer!

[*There is a sudden flash of light: a flare. The* GHOST OF CHRISTMAS PAST *is gone.* SCROOGE *is, for the moment alone onstage. His bed is turned down, across the stage. A small candle burns now in* SCROOGE'*s hand. There is a child's cap in his other*

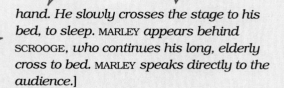

hand. He slowly crosses the stage to his bed, to sleep. MARLEY *appears behind* SCROOGE, *who continues his long, elderly cross to bed.* MARLEY *speaks directly to the audience.*]

MARLEY. Scrooge must sleep now. He must surrender to the irresistible drowsiness caused by the recognition of what was. [*Pauses*] The cap he carries is from ten lives past: his boyhood cap . . . donned atop a hopeful hairy head . . . askew, perhaps, or at a rakish angle. Doffed now in honor of regret. Perhaps even too heavy to carry in his present state of weak remorse . . .

[SCROOGE *drops the cap. He lies atop his bed. He sleeps. To audience*]

He sleeps. For him, there's even more trouble ahead. [*Smiles*] For you? The play house tells me there's hot cider, as should be your anticipation for the specter Christmas Present and Future,

for I promise you both. [*Smiles again*] So, I pray you hurry back to your seats refreshed and ready for a miser—to turn his coat of gray into a blazen Christmas holly-red.

[*A flash of lightning. A clap of thunder. Bats fly. Ghostly music.* MARLEY *is gone.*]

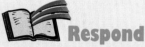

Words to Know

remorse (rih MAWRS) *n.*: Sorrow; regret for previous action

Respond

- How did you feel about Scrooge's behavior? Explain your response.
- In a group, act out what might happen when Scrooge first meets the Ghost of Christmas Present.

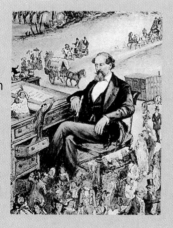

When **Charles Dickens** (1812–1870) was twelve years old, his father went to jail for not paying his debts. Charles had to quit school and go to work in a warehouse pasting labels on bottles of shoe polish. He had to work ten hours a day, six days a week, and then walk home through miles of dangerous streets.

For the rest of his life, he remembered what it was like to be needy. This experience helped shape many

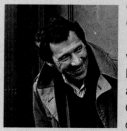

of his stories, including *A Christmas Carol.*

When **Israel Horovitz** (1939–) was twelve, he hated to read books by Charles Dickens. As an adult, he changed his mind. When he adapted *A Christmas Carol* into a play, he decided that his favorite character was Scrooge, who reminded him of his father.

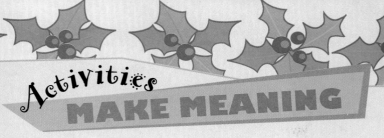

Activities

MAKE MEANING

Explore Your Reading

Look Back (Recall)

1. List the ways in which Scrooge shows that he hates Christmas.

Think It Over (Interpret)

2. Compare and contrast the young Scrooge and the old Scrooge.
3. Why do you think the ghost shows Scrooge "shadows of things that have been"?
4. What hints are there that Scrooge may be changing?

Go Beyond (Apply)

5. What does this play suggest about the way in which people change?

Develop Reading and Literary Skills

Analyze Plot in Drama

As your chart shows, Scrooge faces a variety of conflicts. Conflict is central to the **plot**, or sequence of events in a play. Most plays begin with an **exposition** in which you learn about the setting and characters, and discover the main conflict of the play. In this play, the central conflict relates to Scrooge's stinginess.

Next, the plot moves into the **rising action**, the events of the play that develop a conflict. As Scrooge becomes more upset by his ghostly visitors, your own interest builds. You wonder what the spirits will bring. In the next act, the plot will reach a **climax**, the high point of interest or suspense before the conflicts are solved.

1. Briefly summarize what you learn about the setting, characters, and central conflict in the exposition.
2. Describe Scrooge's conflicts with the other characters.
3. As the action rises, how do Scrooge's conflicts with others turn into struggles within his own mind and heart?

4. Predict how Scrooge's conflicts will be solved in Act II. Support your prediction with evidence from the play.

Ideas for Writing

Act I introduces you to the main characters and the central conflict of the play.

Dramatic Scene Add to Act I by writing a scene that shows Bob Cratchit's job interview with Scrooge. Use the dialogue between them to reveal Scrooge's stinginess.

Personal Letter Suppose that Scrooge's fiancé broke her engagement in a letter rather than in person. Write the letter she would have sent to Scrooge to end their relationship. Make her letter consistent with the scene between them in the play.

Ideas for Projects

Set Design Scripts for plays include descriptions of the sets and props for each scene. Choose a scene in Act I and, using the stage directions, sketch a design for the stage. Also sketch the costumes and props that will bring the play to life. [Art Link]

Invitation to a Holiday Celebration Throughout history, holidays like Christmas have been celebrated with feasts. Research the food and festivities of a holiday feast that you have participated in or know about. Present your results to the class in the form of an invitation. On it include the menu and program of entertainment for the celebration. [Social Studies Link; Art Link]

How Am I Doing?

With a partner, answer these questions:
How did identifying conflicts help me better understand this play?
Which project helped me think about the play? Why?

How can people change in important ways?

Reach Into Your Background

Drama is about change. Imagine how dull it would be to watch characters in a play or a movie if they didn't change at all, if they went on doing the same old things in the same exact ways. That wouldn't be *dramatic.* Watching someone change right before your eyes—a good person going bad or a bad one becoming good—is what keeps you on the edge of your seat.

In a group, explore how characters in drama change by doing one or both of these activities:

• List some ways in which a playwright could show a character changing. How could the playwright make the change more believable?

• As Scrooge, deliver a brief speech that shows you are beginning to change.

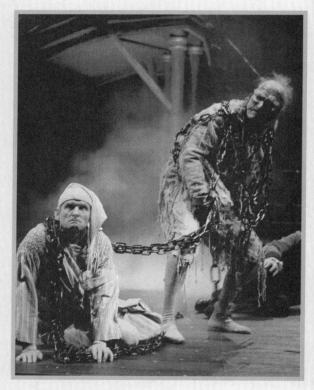

Read Actively
Observe Character Development in Drama

Character development is the means by which playwrights show you characters who grow and change. You can observe such development by noticing differences in a character's appearance, actions, or words. For example, Scrooge's wish to say something to his clerk in Act I, Scene 5, is different from his usual behavior and may be a sign that he is changing. By observing character development, you'll find clues to a play's meaning.

As you read Act II, observe Scrooge's development by jotting down changes in his appearance, actions, and words. Also, think about what these changes say about the play's message.

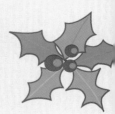

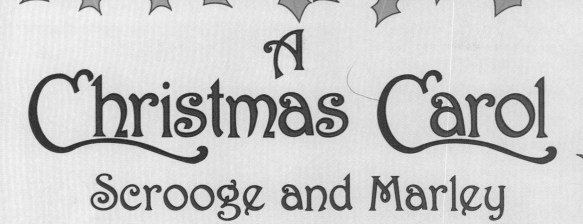

A Christmas Carol
Scrooge and Marley
Act II

ACT II

Scene 1

[*Lights. Choral music is sung. Curtain.* SCROOGE, *in bed, sleeping, in spotlight. We cannot yet see the interior of his room.* MARLEY, *opposite, in spotlight equal to* SCROOGE'S. MARLEY *laughs. He tosses his hand in the air and a flame shoots from it, magically, into the air. There is a thunder clap, and then another; a lightning flash, and then another. Ghostly music plays under. Colors change.* MARLEY'S *spotlight has gone out and now reappears, with* MARLEY *in it, standing next to the bed and the sleeping* SCROOGE. MARLEY *addresses the audience directly.*]

MARLEY. Hear this snoring Scrooge! Sleeping to escape the nightmare that is his waking day. What shall I bring to him now? I'm afraid nothing would astonish old Scrooge now. Not after what he's

seen. Not a baby boy, not a rhinoceros, nor anything in between would astonish Ebenezer Scrooge just now. I can think of nothing . . . [*Suddenly*] that's it! Nothing! [*He speaks confidently.*] I'll have the clock strike one and, when he awakes expecting my second messenger, there will be no one . . . nothing. Then I'll have the bell strike twelve. And then one again . . . and then nothing. Nothing . . . [*Laughs*] nothing will . . . astonish him. I think it will work.

[*The bell tolls one.* SCROOGE *leaps awake.*]

SCROOGE. One! One! This is it: time! [*Looks about the room*] Nothing!

[*The bell tolls midnight.*]

Midnight! How can this be? I'm sleeping backwards.

[*One again*]

Good heavens! One again! I'm sleeping back and forth! [*A pause.* SCROOGE *looks about.*] Nothing! Absolutely nothing!

[*Suddenly, thunder and lightning.* MARLEY *laughs and disappears. The room shakes*

Words to Know

astonish (uh STAHN ish) *v.*: Amaze

and glows. There is suddenly springlike music. SCROOGE *makes a run for the door.*]

MARLEY. Scrooge!

SCROOGE. What?

MARLEY. Stay you put!

SCROOGE. Just checking to see if anyone is in here.

[*Lights and thunder again: more music.* MARLEY *is of a sudden gone. In his place sits the* GHOST OF CHRISTMAS PRESENT—*to be called in the stage directions of the play,* PRESENT—*center of room. Heaped up on the floor, to form a kind of throne, are turkeys, geese, game, poultry, brawn, great joints of meat, suckling pigs, long wreaths of sausages, mince-pies, plum puddings, barrels of oysters, red hot chestnuts, cherry-cheeked apples, juicy oranges, luscious pears, immense twelfth cakes, and seething bowls of punch, that make the chamber dim with their delicious steam. Upon this throne sits* PRESENT, *glorious to see. He bears a torch, shaped as a Horn of Plenty.*[1] SCROOGE *hops out of the door, and then peeks back again into his bedroom.* PRESENT *calls to* SCROOGE.]

PRESENT. Ebenezer Scrooge. Come in, come in! Come in and know me better!

SCROOGE. Hello. How should I call you?

PRESENT. I am the Ghost of Christmas Present. Look upon me.

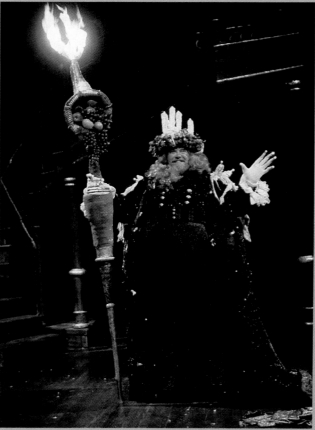

[PRESENT *is wearing a simple green robe. The walls around the room are now covered in greenery, as well. The room seems to be a perfect grove now: leaves of holly, mistletoe and ivy reflect the stage lights. Suddenly, there is a mighty roar of flame in the fireplace and now the hearth burns with a lavish, warming fire. There is an ancient scabbard girdling the* GHOST's *middle, but without sword. The sheath is gone to rust.*]

You have never seen the like of me before?

SCROOGE. Never.

PRESENT. You have never walked forth with younger

---

1. Horn of Plenty: A horn overflowing with fruits, flowers, and grain, standing for wealth and abundance.

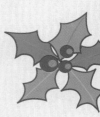

members of my family; my elder brothers born on Christmases past.

SCROOGE. I don't think I have. I'm afraid I've not. Have you had many brothers, Spirit?

PRESENT. More than eighteen hundred.

SCROOGE. A tremendous family to provide for! [PRESENT *stands*] Spirit, conduct me where you will. I went forth last night on compulsion, and learnt a lesson which is working now. Tonight, if you have aught to teach me, let me profit by it.

PRESENT. Touch my robe. [SCROOGE *walks cautiously to* PRESENT *and touches his robe. When he does, lightning flashes, thunder claps, music plays. Blackout*]

Scene 2

[*PROLOGUE:* MARLEY *stands spotlit. L. He speaks directly to the audience.*]

MARLEY. My ghostly friend now leads my living partner through the city's streets.

[*Lights up on* SCROOGE *and* PRESENT]

See them there and hear the music people make when the weather is severe, as it is now.

[*Winter music. Choral group behind scrim, sings. When the song is done and the stage is re-set, the lights will fade up on a row of shops, behind the singers. The* choral group will hum the song they have just completed now and mill about the streets,[2] carrying their dinners to the bakers' shops and restaurants. They will, perhaps, sing about being poor at Christmastime, whatever.]

PRESENT. These revelers, Mr. Scrooge, carry their own dinners to their jobs, where they will work to bake the meals the rich men and women of this city will eat as their Christmas dinners. Generous people these . . . to care for the others, so . . .

[PRESENT *walks among the choral group and a sparkling incense*[3] *falls from his torch on to their baskets, as he pulls the covers off of the baskets. Some of the choral group become angry with each other.*]

MAN #1. Hey, you, watch where you're going.

MAN #2. Watch it yourself, mate!

[PRESENT *sprinkles them directly, they change.*]

MAN #1. I pray go in ahead of me. It's Christmas. You be first!

MAN #2. No, no. I must insist that YOU be first!

MAN #1. All right, I shall be, and gratefully so.

MAN #2. The pleasure is equally mine, for being able to watch you pass, smiling.

---

2. mill about the streets: Walk around aimlessly.

3. incense (IN sens) *n.:* Any various substances that produce a pleasant odor when burned.

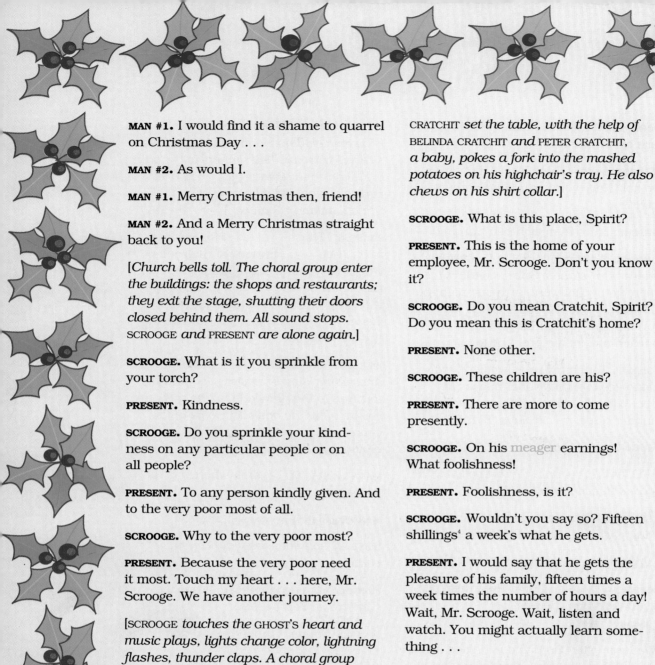

MAN #1. I would find it a shame to quarrel on Christmas Day . . .

MAN #2. As would I.

MAN #1. Merry Christmas then, friend!

MAN #2. And a Merry Christmas straight back to you!

[*Church bells toll. The choral group enter the buildings: the shops and restaurants; they exit the stage, shutting their doors closed behind them. All sound stops.* SCROOGE *and* PRESENT *are alone again.*]

SCROOGE. What is it you sprinkle from your torch?

PRESENT. Kindness.

SCROOGE. Do you sprinkle your kindness on any particular people or on all people?

PRESENT. To any person kindly given. And to the very poor most of all.

SCROOGE. Why to the very poor most?

PRESENT. Because the very poor need it most. Touch my heart . . . here, Mr. Scrooge. We have another journey.

[SCROOGE *touches the* GHOST's *heart and music plays, lights change color, lightning flashes, thunder claps. A choral group appears on the street, singing Christmas carols.*]

Scene 3

[MARLEY *stands spotlit in front of a scrim on which is painted the exterior of* CRATCHIT's *four-roomed house. There is a flash and a clap and* MARLEY *is gone. The lights shift color again, the scrim flies away, and we are in the interior of the* CRATCHIT *family home.* SCROOGE *is there, with the* SPIRIT (PRESENT), *watching* MRS.

CRATCHIT *set the table, with the help of* BELINDA CRATCHIT *and* PETER CRATCHIT, *a baby, pokes a fork into the mashed potatoes on his highchair's tray. He also chews on his shirt collar.*]

SCROOGE. What is this place, Spirit?

PRESENT. This is the home of your employee, Mr. Scrooge. Don't you know it?

SCROOGE. Do you mean Cratchit, Spirit? Do you mean this is Cratchit's home?

PRESENT. None other.

SCROOGE. These children are his?

PRESENT. There are more to come presently.

SCROOGE. On his meager earnings! What foolishness!

PRESENT. Foolishness, is it?

SCROOGE. Wouldn't you say so? Fifteen shillings[4] a week's what he gets.

PRESENT. I would say that he gets the pleasure of his family, fifteen times a week times the number of hours a day! Wait, Mr. Scrooge. Wait, listen and watch. You might actually learn something . . .

MRS. CRATCHIT. What has ever got your precious father then? And your brother, Tiny Tim? And Martha warn't as late last Christmas by half an hour!

[MARTHA *opens the door, speaking to her mother as she does.*]

MARTHA. Here's Martha, now, Mother! [*She laughs. The* CRATCHIT CHILDREN *squeal with delight.*]

---

4. **fifteen shillings:** A small amount of money for a week's work.

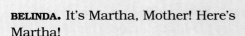

BELINDA. It's Martha, Mother! Here's Martha!

PETER. Marthmama, Marthmama! Hullo!

BELINDA. Hurrah! Martha! Martha! There's such an enormous goose for us, Martha!

MRS. CRATCHIT. Why, bless your heart alive, my dear, how late you are!

MARTHA. We'd a great deal of work to finish up last night, and had to clear away this morning, Mother.

MRS. CRATCHIT. Well, never mind so long as you are come. Sit ye down before the fire, my dear, and have a warm, Lord bless ye!

BELINDA. No, no! There's Father coming. Hide, Martha, hide!

[MARTHA *giggles and hides herself.*]

MARTHA. Where? Here?

PETER. *Hide, hide!*

BELINDA. Not there! *THERE!*

[MARTHA *is hidden.* BOB CRATCHIT *enters, carrying* TINY TIM *atop his shoulder. He wears a* threadbare *and fringeless comforter hanging down in front of him.* TINY TIM *carries small crutches and his small legs are bound in an iron frame brace.*]

BOB and **TINY TIM.** Merry Christmas.

Words to Know

meager (MEE guhr) *adj.*: Of poor quality, small in ammount

threadbare (THRED bayr) *adj.*: Worn; shabby

BOB. Merry Christmas my love, Merry Christmas Peter, Merry Christmas Belinda. Why, where is Martha?

MRS. CRATCHIT. Not coming.

BOB. Not coming: Not coming upon Christmas Day?

MARTHA. [*Pokes head out*] Ohhh, poor Father. Don't be disappointed.

BOB. What's this?

MARTHA. 'Tis I!

BOB. Martha! [*They embrace.*]

TINY TIM. Martha! Martha!

MARTHA. Tiny Tim!

[TINY TIM *is placed in* MARTHA'S *arms.* BELINDA *and* PETER *rush him offstage.*]

BELINDA. Come, brother! You must come hear the pudding singing in the copper.

TINY TIM. The pudding? What flavor have we?

PETER. Plum! Plum!

TINY TIM. Oh, Mother! I love plum!

[*The children exit the stage, giggling.*]

MRS. CRATCHIT. And how did little Tim behave?

BOB. As good as gold, and even better. Somehow he gets thoughtful sitting by himself so much, and thinks the strangest things you ever heard. He told me, coming home, that he hoped people saw him in the church, because he was a cripple, and it might be pleasant to them to remember upon Christmas Day, who made lame beggars walk and blind men see. [*Pauses*] He has the oddest ideas sometimes, but he seems all the while to

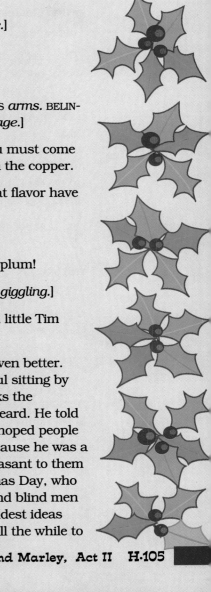

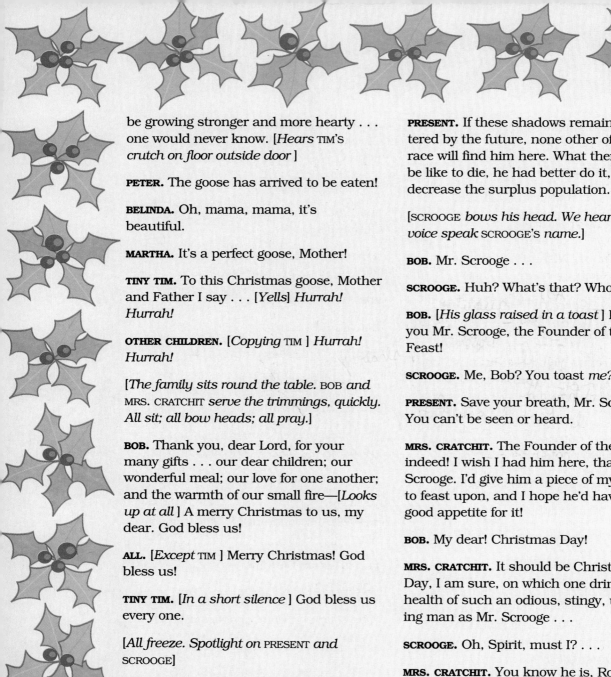

be growing stronger and more hearty . . . one would never know. [*Hears* TIM's *crutch on floor outside door*]

PETER. The goose has arrived to be eaten!

BELINDA. Oh, mama, mama, it's beautiful.

MARTHA. It's a perfect goose, Mother!

TINY TIM. To this Christmas goose, Mother and Father I say . . . [*Yells*] Hurrah! Hurrah!

OTHER CHILDREN. [*Copying* TIM] Hurrah! Hurrah!

[*The family sits round the table.* BOB *and* MRS. CRATCHIT *serve the trimmings, quickly. All sit; all bow heads; all pray.*]

BOB. Thank you, dear Lord, for your many gifts . . . our dear children; our wonderful meal; our love for one another; and the warmth of our small fire—[*Looks up at all*] A merry Christmas to us, my dear. God bless us!

ALL. [*Except* TIM] Merry Christmas! God bless us!

TINY TIM. [*In a short silence*] God bless us every one.

[*All freeze. Spotlight on* PRESENT *and* SCROOGE]

SCROOGE. Spirit, tell me if Tiny Tim will live.

PRESENT. I see a vacant seat . . . in the poor chimney corner, and a crutch without an owner, carefully preserved. If these shadows remain unaltered by the future, the child will die.

SCROOGE. No, no, kind Spirit! Say he will be spared!

PRESENT. If these shadows remain unaltered by the future, none other of my race will find him here. What then? If he be like to die, he had better do it, and decrease the surplus population.

[SCROOGE *bows his head. We hear* BOB's *voice speak* SCROOGE's *name.*]

BOB. Mr. Scrooge . . .

SCROOGE. Huh? What's that? Who calls?

BOB. [*His glass raised in a toast*] I'll give you Mr. Scrooge, the Founder of the Feast!

SCROOGE. Me, Bob? You toast *me?*

PRESENT. Save your breath, Mr. Scrooge. You can't be seen or heard.

MRS. CRATCHIT. The Founder of the Feast, indeed! I wish I had him here, that miser Scrooge. I'd give him a piece of my mind to feast upon, and I hope he'd have a good appetite for it!

BOB. My dear! Christmas Day!

MRS. CRATCHIT. It should be Christmas Day, I am sure, on which one drinks the health of such an odious, stingy, unfeeling man as Mr. Scrooge . . .

SCROOGE. Oh, Spirit, must I? . . .

MRS. CRATCHIT. You know he is, Robert! Nobody knows it better than you do, poor fellow!

BOB. This is Christmas Day, and I should like to drink to the health of the man who employs me and allows me to earn my living and our support and that man is Ebenezer Scrooge . . .

MRS. CRATCHIT. I'll drink to his health for your sake and

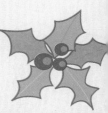

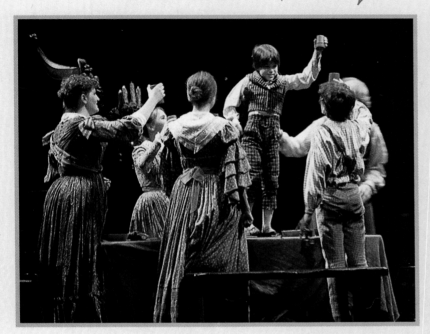

BOB. Martha, will you play the notes on the lute,[5] for Tiny Tim's song.

BELINDA. May I sing, too, Father?

BOB. We'll all sing.

[*They sing a song about a tiny child lost in the snow—probably from Wordsworth's poem.* TIM *sings the lead vocal; all chime in for the chorus. Their song fades under, as* THE GHOST OF CHRISTMAS PRESENT *speaks.*]

the day's, but not for his sake . . . a Merry Christmas and a Happy New Year to you, Mr. Scrooge, wherever you may be this day!

SCROOGE. Just here, kind madam . . . out of sight, out of sight . . .

BOB. Thank you, my dear. Thank you.

SCROOGE. Thank *you*, Bob . . . and Mrs. Cratchit, too. No one else is toasting me, . . . not now . . . not ever. Of that I am sure . . .

BOB. Children . . .

ALL. Merry Christmas to Mr. Scrooge.

BOB. I'll pay you sixpence, Tim, for my favorite song.

TINY TIM. Oh, Father, I'd so love to sing it, but not for pay. This Christmas goose— this feast—you and Mother, my brother and sisters close with me: that's my pay—

PRESENT. Mark my words, Ebenezer Scrooge. I do not present the Cratchits to you because they are a handsome, or brilliant family. They are not handsome. They are not brilliant. They are not well-dressed, or tasteful to the times. Their shoes are not even waterproofed by virtue of money or cleverness spent. So when the pavement is wet, so are the insides of their shoes and the tops of their toes. These are the Cratchits, Mr. Scrooge. They are not highly special. They are happy, grateful, pleased with one another, contented with the time and how it passes. They don't sing very well, do they? But, nonetheless, they do sing . . . [*Pauses*] think of that, Scrooge. Fifteen shillings a week and they do sing . . . hear their song until its end.

SCROOGE. I am listening.

---

5. lute (loot) *n.*: An old-fashioned stringed instrument like a guitar.

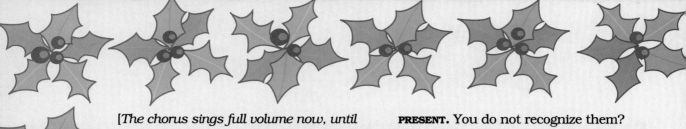

[*The chorus sings full volume now, until . . . the song ends here.*]

Spirit, it must be time for us to take our leave. I feel in my heart that it is . . . that I must think on that which I have seen here . . .

PRESENT. Touch my robe again . . .

[SCROOGE *touches* PRESENT's *robe. The lights fade out on the* CRATCHITS, *who sit, frozen, at the table.* SCROOGE *and* PRESENT *in a spotlight now. Thunder, lightning, smoke. They are gone.*]

Scene 4

[MARLEY *appears D.L. in single spotlight. A storm brews. Thunder and lightning.* SCROOGE *and* PRESENT "*fly*" *past, U. The storm continues, furiously, and, now and again,* SCROOGE *and* PRESENT *will zip past in their travels.* MARLEY *will speak straight out to the audience.*]

MARLEY. The Ghost of Christmas Present, my co-worker in this attempt to turn a miser, flies about now with that very miser, Scrooge, from street to street, and he points out partygoers on their way to Christmas parties. If one were to judge from the numbers of people on their way to friendly gatherings, one might think that no one was left home to give anyone welcome . . . but that's not the case, is it? Every home is expecting company and . . . [*He laughs.*] Scrooge is amazed.

[SCROOGE *and* PRESENT *zip past again. The lights fade up around them. We are in the* NEPHEW's *home, in the living room.* PRESENT *and* SCROOGE *stand watching the* NEPHEW: FRED *and his wife, fixing the fire.*]

SCROOGE. What is this place? We've moved from the mines!

PRESENT. You do not recognize them?

SCROOGE. It is my nephew! . . . and the one he married . . .

[MARLEY *waves his hand and there is a lightning flash. He disappears.*]

FRED. It strikes me as sooooo funny, to think of what he said . . . that Christmas was a humbug, as I live! He believed it!

WIFE. More shame for him, Fred!

FRED. Well, he's a comical old fellow, that's the truth.

WIFE. I have no patience with him.

FRED. Oh, I have! I am sorry for him; I couldn't be angry with him if I tried. Who suffers by his ill whims? Himself, always . . .

SCROOGE. It's me they talk of, isn't it, Spirit?

FRED. Here, wife, consider this. Uncle Scrooge takes it into his head to dislike us, and he won't come and dine with us. What's the consequence?

WIFE. Oh . . . you're sweet to say what I think you're about to say, too, Fred . . .

FRED. What's the consequence? He don't lose much of a dinner by it, I can tell you that!

WIFE. Ooooooo, Fred! Indeed, I think he loses a very good dinner . . . ask my sis-

Words to Know

audible (AW duh buhl) *adj.*: Loud enough to be heard
gnarled (NAHRLD) *adj.*: Knotty and twisted

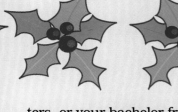
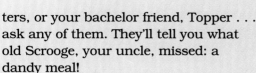

ters, or your bachelor friend, Topper . . . ask any of them. They'll tell you what old Scrooge, your uncle, missed: a dandy meal!

FRED. Well, that's something of a relief, wife. Glad to hear it! [*He hugs his wife. They laugh. They kiss.*] The truth is, he misses much yet. I mean to give him the same chance every year, whether he likes it or not, for I pity him. Nay, he is my only uncle and I feel for the old miser . . . but, I tell you, wife: I see my dear and perfect mother's face on his own wizened cheeks and brow: brother and sister they were, and I cannot erase that from each view of him I take . . .

WIFE. I understand what you say, Fred, and I am with you in your yearly asking. But he never will accept, you know. He never will.

FRED. Well, true, wife. Uncle may rail at Christmas till he dies. I think I shook him some with my visit yesterday . . . [*Laughing*] I refused to grow angry . . . no matter how nasty he became . . . [*Whoops*] It was HE who grew angry, wife! [*They both laugh now.*]

SCROOGE. What he says is true, Spirit . . .

FRED and **WIFE.** Bah, humbug!

FRED. [*Embracing his wife*] There is much laughter in our marriage, wife. It pleases me. You please me . . .

WIFE. And you please me, Fred. You are a good man . . . [*They embrace.*] Come now. We must have a look at the meal . . . our guests will soon arrive . . . my sisters, Topper . . .

FRED. A toast first . . . [*He hands her a glass.*] A toast to Uncle Scrooge . . . [*Fills their glasses*]

WIFE. A toast to him?

FRED. Uncle Scrooge has given us plenty of merriment, I am sure, and it would be ungrateful not to drink to his health. And I say . . . *Uncle Scrooge!*

WIFE. [*Laughing*] You're a proper loon,[6] Fred . . . and I'm a proper wife to you . . . [*She raises her glass.*] Uncle Scrooge! [*They drink. They embrace. They kiss.*]

SCROOGE. Spirit, please, make me visible! Make me audible! I want to talk with my nephew and my niece.

[*Calls out to them. The lights that light the room and* FRED *and* WIFE *fade out.* SCROOGE *and* PRESENT *are alone, spotlit.*]

PRESENT. These shadows are gone to you now, Mr. Scrooge. You may return to them later tonight in your dreams. [*Pauses*] My time grows short, Ebenezer Scrooge. Look you on me! Do you see how I've aged?

SCROOGE. Your hair has gone gray! Your skin, wrinkled! Are spirits' lives so short?

PRESENT. My stay upon this globe is very brief. It ends tonight.

SCROOGE. Tonight?

PRESENT. At midnight. The time is drawing near!

[*Clock strikes 11:45.*]

Hear those chimes? In a quarter hour, my life will have been spent! Look, Scrooge, man. Look you here.

[*Two gnarled baby dolls are taken from* PRESENT'*s skirts.*]

SCROOGE. Who are they?

_____
6. **a proper loon:** A silly person.

PRESENT. They are Man's children, and they cling to me, appealing from their fathers. The boy is Ignorance; the girl is Want. Beware them both, and all of their degree, but most of all beware this boy, for I see that written on his brow which is doom, unless the writing be erased. [*He stretches out his arm. His voice is now amplified: loudly and oddly.*]

SCROOGE. Have they no refuge or resource?

PRESENT. Are there no prisons? Are there no workhouses? [*Twelve chimes*] Are there no prisons? Are there no workhouses?

[*A* PHANTOM, *hooded, appears in dim light, D., opposite.*]

Are there no prisons? Are there no workhouses?

[PRESENT *begins to deliquesce.* SCROOGE *calls after him.*]

SCROOGE. Spirit, I'm frightened! Don't leave me! Spirit!

PRESENT. Prisons? Workhouses? Prisons? Workhouses . . .

[*He is gone.* SCROOGE *is alone now with the* PHANTOM, *who is, of course, the* GHOST OF CHRISTMAS FUTURE. *The* PHANTOM *is shrouded in black. Only its outstretched hand is visible from under his ghostly garment.*]

SCROOGE. Who are you, Phantom? Oh, yes, I think I know you! You are, are you not, the Spirit of Christmas Yet to Come? [*No reply*] And you are about to show me the shadows of the things that have not yet happened, but will happen in time before us. Is that not so, Spirit?

[*The* PHANTOM *allows* SCROOGE *a look at his face. No other reply wanted here. A nervous giggle here*]

Oh, Ghost of the Future, I fear you more than any Specter I have seen! But, as I know that your purpose is to do me good and as I hope to live to be another man from what I was, I am prepared to bear you company.

[FUTURE *does not reply, but for a stiff arm, hand and finger set, pointing forward.*]

Lead on, then, lead on. The night is waning fast, and it is precious time to me. Lead on, Spirit!

[FUTURE *moves away from* SCROOGE *in the same rhythm and motion employed at its arrival.* SCROOGE *falls into the same pattern, a considerable space apart from the* SPIRIT. *In the space between them,* MARLEY *appears. He looks to* FUTURE *and then to* SCROOGE. *He claps his hands. Thunder and lightning. Three* BUSINESSMEN *appear, spotlighted singularly: One is D.L.; one is D.R.; One is U.C. Thus, six points of the stage should now be spotted in light.* MARLEY *will watch this scene from his position, C.* SCROOGE *and* FUTURE *are R. and L. of C.*]

FIRST BUSINESSMAN. Oh, no. I don't know much about it either way. I only know he's dead.

SECOND BUSINESSMAN. When did he die?

FIRST BUSINESSMAN. Last night, I believe.

SECOND BUSINESSMAN. Why, what was the matter with him? I thought he'd never die, really . . .

FIRST BUSINESSMAN. [*Yawning*] Goodness knows, goodness knows . . .

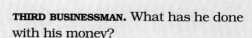

THIRD BUSINESSMAN. What has he done with his money?

SECOND BUSINESSMAN. I haven't heard. Have you?

FIRST BUSINESSMAN. Left it to his Company, perhaps. Money to money; you know the expression . . .

THIRD BUSINESSMAN. He hasn't left it to *me*. That's all I know . . .

FIRST BUSINESSMAN. [*Laughing*] Nor to me . . . [*Looks at* SECOND BUSINESSMAN] You, then? You got his money???

SECOND BUSINESSMAN. [*Laughing*] Me, me, his money? Nooooo! [*They all laugh.*]

THIRD BUSINESSMAN. It's likely to be a cheap funeral, for upon my life, I don't know of a living soul who'd care to venture to it. Suppose we make up a party and volunteer?

SECOND BUSINESSMAN. I don't mind going if a lunch is provided, but I must be fed, if I make one.

FIRST BUSINESSMAN. Well, I am the most disinterested among you, for I never wear black gloves, and I never eat lunch. But I'll offer to go, if anybody else will. When I come to think of it, I'm not all sure that I wasn't his most particular friend; for we used to stop and speak whenever we met. Well, then . . . bye, bye!

SECOND BUSINESSMAN. Bye, bye . . .

THIRD BUSINESSMAN. Bye, bye . . .

[*They glide offstage in three separate directions. Their lights follow them.*]

SCROOGE. Spirit, why did you show me this? Why do you show me businessmen from my streets as they take the death of Jacob Marley. That is a thing past. You are *future!*

[JACOB MARLEY *laughs a long, deep laugh. There is a thunder clap and lightning flash, and he is gone.* SCROOGE *faces* FUTURE, *alone on stage now.* FUTURE *wordlessly stretches out his arm-hand-and-finger-set, pointing into the distance, U. There, above them, Scoundrels "fly" by, half-dressed and slovenly. When this scene has passed, a woman enters the playing area. She is almost at once followed by a second woman; and then a man in faded black; and then, suddenly, an old man, who smokes a pipe. The old man scares the other three. They laugh, anxious.*]

FIRST WOMAN. Look here, old Joe, here's a chance! If we haven't all three met here without meaning it!

OLD JOE. You couldn't have met in a better place. Come into the parlor. You were made free of it long ago, you know; and the other two an't strangers [*He stands; shuts a door. Shrieking*] We're all suitable to our calling. We're well matched. Come into the parlor. Come into the parlor . . .

[*They follow him D.* SCROOGE *and* FUTURE *are now in their midst, watching: silent. A truck comes in on which is set a small wall with fireplace and a screen of rags, etc. All props for the scene.*]

Let me just rake this fire over a bit . . .

[*He does. He trims his lamp with the stem of his pipe. The* FIRST WOMAN *throws a large bundle on to the floor. She sits beside it, crosslegged, defiantly.*]

FIRST WOMAN. What odds then? What odds, Mrs. Dilber? Every person has a

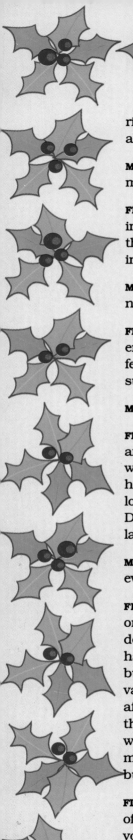

right to take care of themselves. HE always did!

MRS. DILBER. That's true indeed! No man more so!

FIRST WOMAN. Why, then, don't stand staring as if you was afraid, woman! Who's the wiser? We're not going to pick holes in each other's coats, I suppose?

MRS. DILBER. No, indeed! We should hope not!

FIRST WOMAN. Very well, then! That's enough. Who's the worse for the loss of a few things like these? Not a dead man, I suppose?

MRS. DILBER. [*Laughing*] No, indeed!

FIRST WOMAN. If he wanted to keep 'em after he was dead, the wicked old screw, why wasn't he natural in his lifetime? If he had been, he'd have had somebody to look after him when he was struck with Death, instead of lying gasping out his last there, alone by himself.

MRS. DILBER. It's the truest word that was ever spoke. It's a judgment on him.

FIRST WOMAN. I wish it were a heavier one, and it should have been, you may depend on it, if I could have laid my hands on anything else. Open that bundle, old Joe, and let me know the value of it. Speak out plain. I'm not afraid to be the first, nor afraid for them to see it. We knew pretty well that we were helping ourselves, before we met here, I believe. It's no sin. Open the bundle, Joe.

FIRST MAN. No, no, my dear! I won't think of letting you being the first to show what you've . . . earned . . . earned from this. I throw in mine. [*He takes a bundle from his shoulder, turns it upside down, and empties its contents out on to the floor.*] It's not very extensive, see . . . seals . . . a pencil case . . . sleeve buttons . . .

MRS. DILBER. Nice sleeve buttons, though . . .

FIRST MAN. Not bad, not bad . . . a brooch there . . .

OLD JOE. Not really valuable, I'm afraid. . .

FIRST MAN. How much, old Joe?

OLD JOE. [*Writing on the wall with chalk*] A pitiful lot, really. Ten and six and not a six-pence more!

FIRST MAN. You're not serious!

OLD JOE. That's your account and I wouldn't give another sixpence if I was to be boiled for not doing it. Who's next?

MRS. DILBER. Me! [*Dumps out contents of her bundle*] Sheets, towels, silver spoons, silver sugar-tongs . . . some boots . . .

OLD JOE. [*Writing on wall*] I always give too much to the ladies. It's a weakness of mine and that's the way I ruin myself. Here's your total comin' up . . . two pounds-ten . . . if you asked me for another penny, and made it an open question, I'd repent of being so liberal and knock off half-a-crown.

FIRST WOMAN. And now do MY bundle, Joe.

OLD JOE. [*Kneeling to open knots on her bundle*] So many knots, madam . . . [*He drags out large curtains: dark*] What do you call this? Bed curtains!

FIRST WOMAN. [*Laughing*] Ah, yes, bed curtains!

OLD JOE. You don't mean to say you took 'em down, rings and all, with him lying there?

FIRST WOMAN. Yes, I did, why not?

OLD JOE. You were born to make your fortune and you'll certainly do it.

FIRST WOMAN. I certainly shan't hold my hand, when I can get anything in it by reaching it out, for the sake of such a man as he was, I promise you, Joe. Don't drop that lamp oil on those blankets, now!

OLD JOE. His blankets?

FIRST WOMAN. Whose else's do you think? He isn't likely to catch cold without 'em, I daresay.

OLD JOE. I hope that he didn't die of anything catching? Eh?

FIRST WOMAN. Don't you be afraid of that. I ain't so fond of his company that I'd loiter about him for such things if he did. Ah! You may look through that shirt till your eyes ache, but you won't find a hole in it, nor a threadbare place. It's the best he had, and a fine one, too. They'd have wasted it, if it hadn't been for me.

OLD JOE. What do you mean "They'd have wasted it"?

FIRST WOMAN. Putting it on him to be buried in, to be sure. Somebody was fool enough to do it, but I took it off again . . . [*She laughs, as do they all, nervously.*] If calico[7] ain't good enough for such a purpose, it isn't good enough then for anything. It's quite as becoming to the body. He can't look uglier than he did in that one!

------
7. **calico** (KAL uh koh) *n.*: A coarse and cheap cloth.

SCROOGE. [*A low-pitched moan emits from his mouth; from the bones.*] OOOOOOOoo oooOOOOOooooOOOOOOOOoooooOOO OOOoooooOO!

OLD JOE. One pound six for the lot. [*He produces a small flannel bag filled with money. He divvies it out. He continues to pass around the money as he speaks. All are laughing.*] That's the end of it, you see! He frightened every one away from him while he was alive, to profit us when he was dead! Hah ha ha!

ALL. HAHAHAHAhahahahahahah!

SCROOGE. OOOoooOOOoooOOOoooOOO oooOOoooOOoooOOOooo! [*He screams at them.*] Obscene demons! Why not market the corpse itself, as sell its trimming??? [*Suddenly*] Oh, Spirit, I see it, I see it! This unhappy man—this stripped-bare corpse . . . could very well be my own. My life holds parallel! My life ends that way now!

[SCROOGE *backs into something in the dark behind his spotlight.* SCROOGE *looks at* FUTURE, *who points to the corpse.* SCROOGE *pulls back the blanket. The corpse is, of course,* SCROOGE, *who screams. He falls aside the bed; weeping.*]

Spirit, this is a fearful place. In leaving it, I shall not leave its lesson, trust me. Let us go!

[FUTURE *points to the corpse.*]

Spirit, let me see some tenderness connected with a death, or that dark chamber, which we just left now, Spirit, will be forever present to me.

[FUTURE *spreads his robes again. Thunder and lightning. Lights up, U., in the Cratchit home setting.* MRS. CRATCHIT *and her daughters, sewing*]

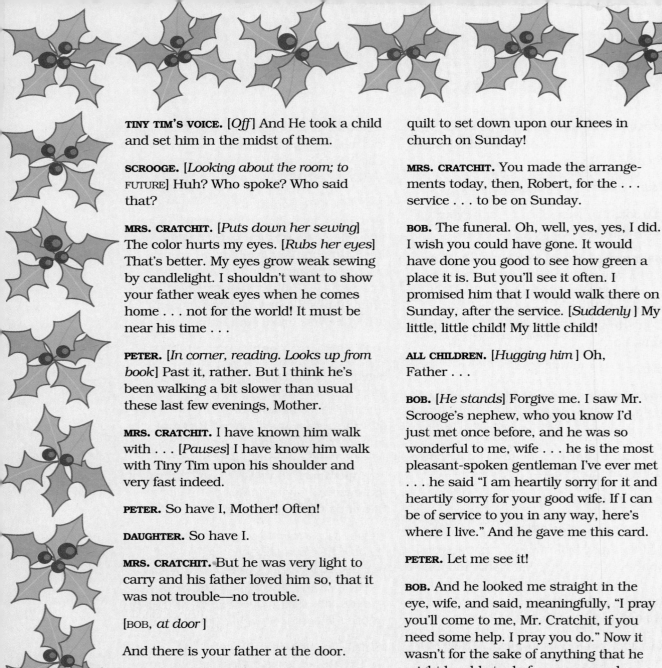

TINY TIM'S VOICE. [*Off*] And He took a child and set him in the midst of them.

SCROOGE. [*Looking about the room; to* FUTURE] Huh? Who spoke? Who said that?

MRS. CRATCHIT. [*Puts down her sewing*] The color hurts my eyes. [*Rubs her eyes*] That's better. My eyes grow weak sewing by candlelight. I shouldn't want to show your father weak eyes when he comes home . . . not for the world! It must be near his time . . .

PETER. [*In corner, reading. Looks up from book*] Past it, rather. But I think he's been walking a bit slower than usual these last few evenings, Mother.

MRS. CRATCHIT. I have known him walk with . . . [*Pauses*] I have know him walk with Tiny Tim upon his shoulder and very fast indeed.

PETER. So have I, Mother! Often!

DAUGHTER. So have I.

MRS. CRATCHIT. But he was very light to carry and his father loved him so, that it was not trouble—no trouble.

[BOB, *at door*]

And there is your father at the door.

[BOB CRATCHIT *enters. He wears a comforter. He is cold, forlorn.*]

PETER. Father!

BOB. Hello, wife, children . . .

[*The daughter weeps; turns away from* CRATCHIT.]

Children! How good to see you all! And you, wife. And look at this sewing! I've no doubt, with all your industry, we'll have a quilt to set down upon our knees in church on Sunday!

MRS. CRATCHIT. You made the arrangements today, then, Robert, for the . . . service . . . to be on Sunday.

BOB. The funeral. Oh, well, yes, yes, I did. I wish you could have gone. It would have done you good to see how green a place it is. But you'll see it often. I promised him that I would walk there on Sunday, after the service. [*Suddenly*] My little, little child! My little child!

ALL CHILDREN. [*Hugging him*] Oh, Father . . .

BOB. [*He stands*] Forgive me. I saw Mr. Scrooge's nephew, who you know I'd just met once before, and he was so wonderful to me, wife . . . he is the most pleasant-spoken gentleman I've ever met . . . he said "I am heartily sorry for it and heartily sorry for your good wife. If I can be of service to you in any way, here's where I live." And he gave me this card.

PETER. Let me see it!

BOB. And he looked me straight in the eye, wife, and said, meaningfully, "I pray you'll come to me, Mr. Cratchit, if you need some help. I pray you do." Now it wasn't for the sake of anything that he might be able to do for us, so much as for his kind way. It seemed as if he had known our Tiny Tim and felt with us.

MRS. CRATCHIT. I'm sure that he's a good soul.

BOB. You would be surer of it, my dear, if you saw and spoke to him. I shouldn't be at all surprised, if he got Peter a situation.

MRS. CRATCHIT. Only hear that, Peter!

MARTHA. And then, Peter will be keeping company with someone and setting up for himself!

PETER. Get along with you!

BOB. It's just as likely as not, one of these days, though there's plenty of time for that, my dear. But however and whenever we part from one another, I am sure we shall none of us forget poor Tiny Tim—shall we?—or this first parting that was among us?

ALL CHILDREN. Never, Father, never!

BOB. And when we recollect how patient and mild he was, we shall not quarrel easily among ourselves, and forget poor Tiny Tim in doing it.

ALL CHILDREN. No, Father, never!

LITTLE BOB. I am very happy, I am, I am, I am very happy.

[BOB *kisses his little son, as does* MRS. CRATCHIT, *as do the other children. The family is set now in one sculptural embrace. The lighting fades to a gentle pool of light, tight on them.*]

SCROOGE. Specter, something informs me that our parting moment is at hand. I know it, but I know not how I know it.

[FUTURE *points to the other side of the stage. Lights out on Cratchits.* FUTURE *moves slowly, gliding.* SCROOGE *follows.* FUTURE *points opposite.* FUTURE *leads* SCROOGE *to a wall and a tombstone. He points to the stone.*]

Am *I* that man those ghoulish parasites[8] so gloated over? [*Pauses*] Before I draw nearer to that stone to which you point, answer me one question. Are these the shadows of things that will be, or the shadows of things that MAY be, only?

[FUTURE *points to the gravestone.* MARLEY *appears in light well U. He points to grave as well. Gravestone turns front and grows to ten feet high. Words upon it: EBENEZER SCROOGE. Much smoke billows now from the grave. Choral music here.* SCROOGE *stands looking up at gravestone.* FUTURE *does not at all reply in mortals'*

---

8. ghoulish parasites (GOOL ish PAR uh sì ts): The man and women who stole and divided Scrooge's goods after he died.

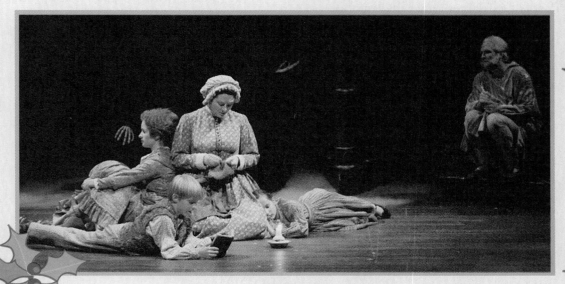

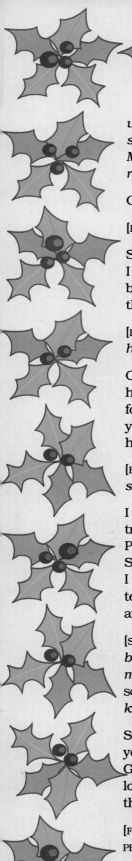

words, but points once more to the grave-stone. The stone undulates and glows. Music plays, beckoning SCROOGE. SCROOGE reeling in terror]

Oh, no. Spirit! Oh, no, no!

[FUTURE's *finger still pointing*]

Spirit! Hear me! I am not the man I was. I will not be the man I would have been but for this intercourse. Why show me this, if I am past all hope?

[FUTURE *considers* SCROOGE's *logic. His hand wavers.*]

Oh, Good Spirit, I see by your wavering hand that your good nature intercedes for me and pities me. Assure me that I yet may change these shadows that you have shown me by an altered life!

[FUTURE's *hand trembles; pointing has stopped.*]

I will honor Christmas in my heart and try to keep it all the year. I will live in the Past, the Present, and the Future. The Spirits of all Three shall strive within me. I will not shut out the lessons that they teach. Oh, tell me that I may sponge away the writing that is upon this stone!

[SCROOGE *makes a desperate stab at grabbing* FUTURE's *hand. He holds it firm for a moment, but* FUTURE, *stronger than* SCROOGE, *pulls away.* SCROOGE *is on his knees, praying.*]

Spirit, dear Spirit, I am praying before you. Give me a sign that all is possible. Give me a sign that all hope for me is not lost. Oh, Spirit, kind Spirit, I beseech thee: give me a sign . . .

[FUTURE *deliquesces, slowly, gently. The* PHANTOM's *hood and robe drop gracefully*

to the ground in a small heap. Music in. There is nothing in them. They are mortal cloth. The Spirit is elsewhere. SCROOGE *has his sign.* SCROOGE *is alone. Tableau. The lights fade to black.*]

Scene 5

[*The end of it.* MARLEY, *spotlighted, opposite* SCROOGE, *in his bed, spotlighted.* MARLEY *speaks to audience, directly.*]

MARLEY. [*He smiles at* SCROOGE.] The firm of Scrooge and Marley is doubly blessed; two misers turned; one, alas, in Death, too late; but the other miser turned in Time's penultimate nick.[9] Look you on my friend, Ebenezer Scrooge . . .

SCROOGE. [*Scrambling out of bed; reeling in delight*] I will live in the Past, in the Present, and in the Future! The Spirits of all Three shall strive within me!

MARLEY. [*He points and moves closer to* SCROOGE's *bed.*] Yes, Ebenezer, the bed-post is your own. Believe it! Yes, Ebenezer, the room is your own. Believe it!

SCROOGE. Oh, Jacob Marley! Wherever you are, Jacob, know ye that I praise you for this! I praise you . . . and heaven . . . and Christmastime! [*Kneels facing away from* MARLEY] I say it to ye on my knees, Old Jacob, on my knees! [*He touches his bed curtains.*] Not torn down. My bed curtains are not at all torn down! Rings and all, here they are! They are here: I

---

9. in Time's penultimate nick: Just at the last moment.

Words to Know

dispelled (dis PELD) *v.*: Scattered and driven away, made to vanish; dispelled

am here: the shadows of things that would have been, may now be dispelled. They will be, Jacob! I know they will be! [*He chooses clothing for the day. He tries different pieces of clothing and settles, perhaps on a dress suit, plus a cape of the bed clothing: something of color.*] I am light as a feather, I am happy as an angel, I am as merry as a schoolboy. [*Yells out window and then out to audience*] Merry Christmas to everybody! Merry Christmas to everybody! A Happy New Year to all the world! Hallo here! Whoop! Whoop! Hallo! Hallo! I don't know what day of the month it is! I don't care! I don't know anything! I'm quite a baby! I don't care! I don't care a fig! I'd much rather be a baby than be an old wreck like me or Marley! (Sorry, Jacob, wherever ye be!) Hallo! Hallo there!

[*Church bells chime in Christmas Day. A small boy, named* ADAM, *is seen now D.R., as a light fades up on him.*]

Hey, you boy! What's today? What day of the year is it?

ADAM. Today, sir? Why, it's Christmas Day!

SCROOGE. It's Christmas Day, is it? Whoop! Well, I haven't missed it after all, have I? The Spirits did all they did in one night. They can do anything they like, right? Of course they can! Of course they can!

ADAM. Excuse me, sir?

SCROOGE. Huh? Oh, yes, of course, what's your name, lad?

[SCROOGE *and* ADAM *will play their scene from their own spotlights.*]

> **ADAM.** Adam, sir.

SCROOGE. Adam! What a fine, strong name! Do you know the poulterer's[10] in the next street but one, at the corner?

ADAM. I certainly should hope I know him, sir!

SCROOGE. A remarkable boy! An intelligent boy! Do you know whether the poulterer's have sold the prize turkey that was hanging up there? I don't mean the little prize turkey, Adam. I mean the big one!

ADAM. What, do you mean the one they've got that's as big as me?

SCROOGE. I mean, the turkey the size of Adam: that's the bird!

ADAM. It's hanging there now, sir.

SCROOGE. It is? Go and buy it! No, no, I am absolutely in earnest. Go and buy it and tell 'em to bring it here, so that I may give them the directions to where I want it delivered, as a gift. Come back here with the man, Adam, and I'll give you a shilling. Come back here with him in less than five minutes, and I'll give you half-a-crown!

ADAM. Oh, my sir! Don't let my brother in on this.

[ADAM *runs offstage.* MARLEY *smiles.*]

MARLEY. An act of kindness is like the first green grape of summer: one leads to another and another and another. It would take a queer man indeed to not follow an act of kindness with an act of kindness. One simply whets the tongue for more . . . the taste of kindness is too too sweet. Gifts—goods—are lifeless. But

---

10. poulterer's (POHL tuhr erz) *n.:* A British world for a store that sells chickens, turkeys, and geese.

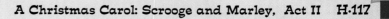

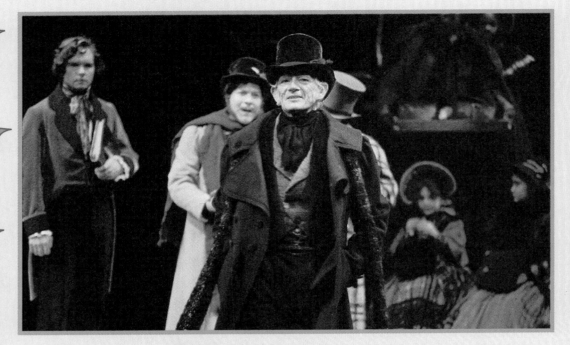

the gift of goodness one feels in the giving is full of life. It . . . is . . . a . . . wonder.

[*Pauses: moves closer to* SCROOGE, *who is totally occupied with his dressing, and arranging of his room and his day. He is making lists, etc.* MARLEY *reaches out to* SCROOGE.]

ADAM. [*Calling, off*] I'm here! I'm here!

[ADAM *runs on with a man, who carries an enormous turkey.*]

Here I am, sir, Three minutes flat! A world record! I've got the poultryman and he's got the poultry! [*He pants, out of breath.*] I have earned my prize, sir, if I live . . .

[*He holds his heart, playacting.* SCROOGE *goes to him and embraces him.*]

SCROOGE. You are truly a champion, Adam . . .

MAN. Here's the bird you ordered, sir . . .

SCROOGE. *Oh, my, MY!!!* Look at the size of that turkey, will you! He never could have stood upon his legs, that bird! He would have snapped them off in a minute, like sticks of sealingwax! Why you'll never be able to carry that bird to Camden-Town. I'll give you money for a cab . . .

MAN. Camden-Town's where it's goin', sir?

SCROOGE. Oh, I didn't tell you? Yes, I've written the precise address down just here on this . . . [*Hands paper to him*] Bob Cratchit's house. Now he's not to know who sends him this. Do you understand me? Not a word . . . [*Handing out money and chuckling*]

MAN. I understand, sir, not a word.

SCROOGE. Good. There you go then . . . this is for the turkey . . . [*Chuckle*] and this is for the taxi. [*Chuckle*] . . . and this is for your world-record run, Adam . . .

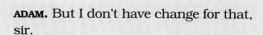

ADAM. But I don't have change for that, sir.

SCROOGE. Then keep it, my lad. It's Christmas!

ADAM. [*He kisses* SCROOGE's *cheek, quickly.*] Thank you, sir. Merry, Merry Christmas! [*He runs off.*]

MAN. And you've given me a bit overmuch here, too, sir . . .

SCROOGE. Of course I have, sir. It's Christmas!

MAN. Oh, well, thanking you, sir. I'll have this bird to Mr. Cratchit and his family in no time, sir. Don't you worry none about that. Merry Christmas to you, sir, and a very happy New Year, too . . .

[*The man exits.* SCROOGE *walks in a large circle about the stage, which is now gently lit. A chorus sings Christmas music far in the distance. Bells chime as well, far in the distance. A gentlewoman enters and passes.* SCROOGE *is on the streets now.*]

SCROOGE. Merry Christmas, madam . . .

WOMAN. Merry Christmas, sir . . .

[*The portly businessman from the first act enters.*]

SCROOGE. Merry Christmas, sir.

PORTLY MAN. Merry Christmas, sir.

SCROOGE. Oh, you! My dear sir! How do you do? I do hope that you succeeded yesterday! It was very kind of you. A Merry Christmas.

PORTLY MAN. Mr. Scrooge?

SCROOGE. Yes, Scrooge is my name though I'm afraid you may not find it very pleasant.

Allow me to ask your pardon. And will you have the goodness to— [*He whispers into the man's ear.*]

PORTLY MAN. Lord bless me! My dear Mr. Scrooge, are you *serious!?!*

SCROOGE. If you please. Not a farthing[11] less. A great many back payments are included in it, I assure you. Will you do me that favor?

PORTLY MAN. My dear sir, I don't know what to say to such munifi—

SCROOGE. [*Cutting him off*] Don't say anything, please. Come and see me. Will you?

PORTLY MAN. I will! I will! Oh I will, Mr. Scrooge! It will be my pleasure!

SCROOGE. Thank'ee, I am much obliged to you. I thank you fifty times. Bless you!

[PORTLY MAN *passes offstage, perhaps by moving backwards.* SCROOGE *now comes to the room of his* NEPHEW *and* NIECE. *He stops at the door, begins to knock on it, loses his courage, tries again, loses his courage again, tries again, fails again, and then backs off and runs at the door, causing a tremendous bump against it. The* NEPHEW *and* NIECE *are startled.* SCROOGE, *poking head into room*]

Fred!

NEPHEW. Why, bless my soul! Who's that?

NEPHEW and **NIECE.** [*Together*] How now? Who goes?

SCROOGE. It's I. Your Uncle Scrooge.

NIECE. Dear heart alive!

---

11. farthing (FAHR thing) *n.*: A small British coin.

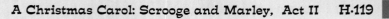

SCROOGE. I have come to dinner. May I come in, Fred?

NEPHEW. *May you come in???!!!* With such pleasure for me you may, Uncle!!! What a treat!

NIECE. What a treat, Uncle Scrooge! Come in, come in.

[They embrace a shocked and delighted SCROOGE. FRED *calls into the other room.]*

NEPHEW. Come in here, everybody, and meet my Uncle Scrooge! He's come for our Christmas party!

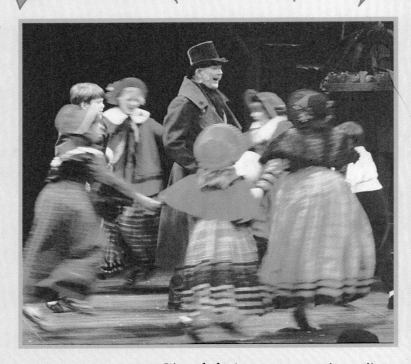

[Music in. Lighting here indicates that day is gone to night and gone to day again. It is early, early morning. SCROOGE *walks alone from the party, exhausted, to his offices, opposite side of the stage. He opens his offices. The offices are as they were at the start of the play.* SCROOGE *seats himself with his door wide open so that he can see into the tank, as he awaits* CRATCHIT, *who enters, head down, full of guilt.* CRATCHIT *starts writing almost before he sits.]*

SCROOGE. What do you mean by coming in here at this time of day, a full eighteen minutes late, Mr. Cratchit? Hallo, sir? Do you hear me?

BOB. I am very sorry, sir. I *am* behind my time.

SCROOGE. You are? Yes, I certainly think you are. Step this way, sir, if you please . . .

BOB. It's only but once a year, sir . . . it shall not be repeated. I was making rather merry yesterday and into the night . . .

SCROOGE. Now, I'll tell you what, Cratchit. I am not going to stand this sort of thing any longer. And therefore . . .

[He stands and pokes his finger into BOB'S *chest.]*

I am . . . about . . . to . . . raise . . . your salary.

BOB. Oh, no, sir, I . . . *[Realizes]* what did you say , sir?

SCROOGE. A Merry Christmas, Bob . . . *[He claps* BOB'S *back.]* A merrier Christmas, Bob, my good fellow! than I have given you for many a year. I'll raise your salary and endeavor to assist your struggling family and we will discuss your affairs this very afternoon over a bowl of smoking bishop.[12] Bob! Make up the fires and buy another coal scuttle before you dot another i, Bob. It's too cold in this place! We need warmth and cheer, Bob Cratchit! Do you hear me? DO . . . YOU. . . HEAR . . . ME?

[BOB CRATCHIT *stands, smiles at* SCROOGE. BOB CRATCHIT *faints. Blackout. As the main lights black out, a spotlight appears on* SCROOGE. C. *Another on* MARLEY. *He talks directly to the audience.*]

MARLEY. Scrooge was better than his word. He did it all and infinitely more; and to Tiny Tim, who did NOT die, he was a second father. He became as good a friend, as good a master, as good a man, as the good old city knew, or any other good old city, town, or borough in the good old world. And it was always said of him that he knew how to keep

12. **smoking bishop:** A hot, sweet, orange-flavored drink.

Christmas well, if any man alive possessed the knowledge. [*Pauses*] May that be truly said of us, and all of us. And so, as Tiny Tim observed . . .

TINY TIM. [*Atop* SCROOGE's *shoulder*] God Bless Us, Every One . . .

[*Lights up on the chorus, singing final Christmas Song.* SCROOGE *and* MARLEY *and all spirits and other characters of the play join in. When the song is over, the lights fade to black.*]

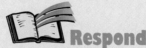

Respond

- Would this play have worked as well without ghosts? Why or why not?
- Would knowing what you'll be like in ten years change the way you act now? In a small group, discuss the pros and cons of having such information.

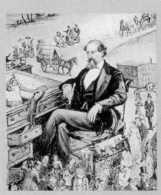

Charles Dickens
Quotation:
"I have endeavoured, in this ghostly little book, to raise the Ghost of an Idea, which shall not put my readers out of humour with themselves, with each other, with the season, or with me. May it haunt their houses pleasantly . . .
Their faithful friend and servant,
Charles Dickens."
from *A Christmas Carol,* by Charles Dickens

Israel Horowitz
Quotation:
"Sometimes, I use my writing to relive the past . . . re-do history . . . get it right. (I still call this sort of work 'righting'.)"

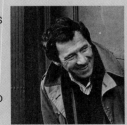

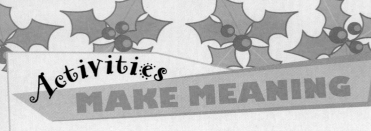

Activities
MAKE MEANING

Explore Your Reading

Look Back (Recall)

1. What do the Ghosts of Christmas Present and Future show to Scrooge?

Think It Over (Interpret)

2. In Scene 4 Scrooge says, "Spirit, please, make me visible! . . . I want to talk with my nephew and my niece!" What would he have said if he could?
3. What does this wish to speak show about him?
4. How does Marley's speech about "[a]n act of kindness" in Scene 5 summarize what has happened to Scrooge?

Go Beyond (Apply)

5. Dickens wrote *A Christmas Carol* in the 1800's. How does the story apply to us today?

Develop Reading and Literary Skills

Understand Character Development and Theme

You've observed how the playwright uses techniques of **character development** to show how Scrooge grows. These techniques include changes in Scrooge's appearance, actions, and words. For example, when he wakes up on Christmas morning, he does something the old Scrooge would never have done. He yells out the window, "Merry Christmas to everybody!"

Character development in drama is often a clue to a play's **theme,** or central idea about life. As a changed man, Scrooge can serve as an example for all of us.

1. Find two ways in which the playwright shows you Scrooge in the process of changing. Explain each choice.
2. Find an additional example from the play that shows Scrooge *has* changed. Explain.
3. How is Scrooge's change a key to the play's meaning?

Ideas for Writing

A good drama can spark your imagination in many ways.

Double Eulogy Scrooge has just passed away. You have been chosen to write his eulogy, a speech in praise of someone who has died. First imagine that he didn't change his ways, so you must write a eulogy for the old Scrooge. Then write another eulogy for the changed Scrooge.

Casting Memo Write a memo to the director of a new production of *A Christmas Carol.* Suggest actors for the major parts and include persuasive reasons for your choices.

Ideas for Projects

History of Christmas Research how people celebrated Christmas from the earliest times through the late 1800's. Present your findings to your classmates. [Social Studies Link]

Holiday Research Learn about holidays that resemble Christmas in their emphasis on giving. Study holidays from as many different cultures as possible and write brief descriptions of each for your classmates. [Social Studies Link]

Character Profile Ask your school guidance counselor how accurate the play is as a profile of someone who changes. Have the guidance counselor speak about these issues to your classmates, or present the findings yourself.

How Am I Doing?

Answer the following questions in your journal:
How did observing Scrooge's change help me understand the theme of the play?

What does Dickens say in this play about our responsibility to others and doing what's right? What do I believe about my responsibility to others?

What Matters Most?

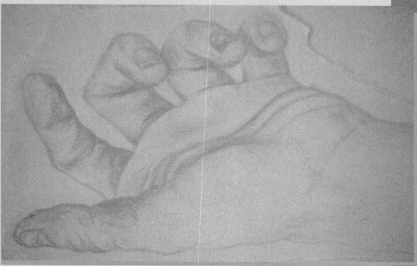

Student Art *Untitled* Robert Wall
Overton High School, Memphis, Tennessee

Grandpa's Hand

Student Writing Juli Peterson, Libby Middle School
Spokane, Washington

I was only about four when he held his hand out to me. I took it in mine and we walked. Then I asked him, "Grandpa, why do you have so many wrinkles on your hand?"

He laughed and said, "Well, Grandson, that's a grand question!" He was silent for a moment. He must have been thinking.

This was his answer: "Each one of these wrinkles stands for a trouble I've had through my years, and each of the troubles I've lived through."

I looked at his other hand. "But Grandpa," I said. "How come you have even more on that one?"

"Those are for all the glories and joys in my life."

"Grandpa," I said. "May I count them?"

What is your most important treasure?

Reach Into Your Background

As a child, you probably had some special treasure — a toy truck, a stuffed animal, or an old baseball. Today, that item might make you smile, but other things have probably become more important to you. Some of today's treasures may be material objects like a guitar, or a camera. Others may be less tangible things, like friendship, success, and achievement.

Consider what matters most to you by trying one or both of these activities:

- Write a journal entry about your personal treasures, explaining why they are important to you.
- With a small group, play a pantomime game in which each of you uses movements and expressions—but not words—to describe a "treasure." Have other group members guess what it is.

Read Actively
Identify Details of Setting

Sometimes the memory of a particular place and time can be a treasure. The **setting**, or place and time, of a story can also be important. Details of the setting might include anything from a character's coat to the color of a distant mountain range. By identifying these details, you will feel more at home in the story's world. You will also see how that world influences the characters.

In this story, weather and an abandoned building are two crucial details of the setting. Identify others by filling in a cluster diagram like this one.

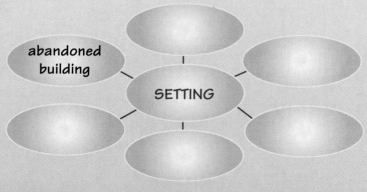

abandoned building

SETTING

The Treasure of
Lemon Brown
Walter Dean Myers

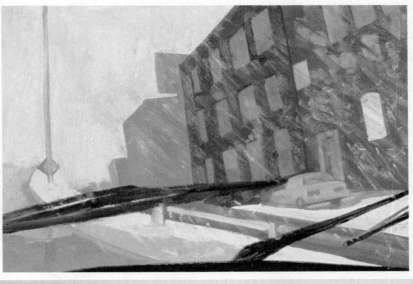

Snowy Street Scene
Catherine Redmond
Courtesy of the artist

The dark sky, filled with angry, swirling clouds, reflected Greg Ridley's mood as he sat on the stoop of his building. His father's voice came to him again, first reading the letter the principal had sent to the house, then lecturing endlessly about his poor efforts in math.

"I had to leave school when I was thirteen," his father had said, "that's a year younger than you are now. If I'd had half the chances that you have, I'd . . ."

Greg had sat in the small, pale green kitchen listening, knowing the lecture would end with his father saying he couldn't play ball with the Scorpions. He had asked his father the week before, and his father had said it depended on his next report card. It wasn't often the Scorpions took on new players, especially fourteen-year-olds, and this was a chance of a lifetime for Greg. He hadn't been allowed to play high school ball, which he had really wanted to do, but playing for the Community Center team was the next best thing. Report cards were due in a week, and Greg had been hoping for the best. But the principal had ended the suspense early when she sent that letter saying Greg would probably fail math if he didn't spend more time studying.

"And you want to play *basketball*?" His father's brows knitted over deep brown eyes. "That must be some kind of a joke. Now you just get into your room and hit those books."

That had been two nights before. His father's words, like the distant thunder that now echoed through the streets of Harlem, still rumbled softly in his ears.

It was beginning to cool. Gusts of wind made bits of paper dance between the parked cars. There was a flash of nearby lightning, and soon large drops of rain splashed onto his jeans. He stood to go upstairs, thought of the lecture that probably awaited him if he did anything except shut himself in his room with his math book, and started walking down the street instead. Down the block there was an old tenement[1] that had been abandoned for some months. Some of the guys had held an impromptu checker tournament there the week before, and Greg had noticed that the door, once boarded over, had been slightly ajar.

Pulling his collar up as high as he could, he checked for traffic and made a dash across the street. He reached the house just as another flash of lightning changed the night to day for an instant, then returned the graffiti-scarred building to the grim shadows. He vaulted over the outer stairs and pushed tentatively on the door. It was open, and he let himself in.

The inside of the building was dark except for the dim light that filtered through the dirty windows from the street-lamps. There was a room a few feet from the door,

📖 **Read Actively**

Visualize the inside of the old tenement.

and from where he stood at the entrance, Greg could see a squarish patch of light on the floor. He entered the room, frowning at the musty smell. It was a large room that might have been someone's parlor at one time. Squinting, Greg could see an old table on its side against one wall, what looked like a pile of rags or a torn mattress in the corner, and a couch, with one side broken, in front of the window.

He went to the couch. The side that wasn't broken was comfortable enough, though a little creaky. From the spot he could see the blinking neon sign over the bodega[2] on the corner. He sat awhile, watching the sign blink first green then red, allowing his mind to drift to the Scorpions, then to his father. His father had been a postal worker for all Greg's life, and was proud of it, often telling Greg how hard he had worked to pass the test. Greg had heard the story too many times to be interested now.

For a moment Greg thought he heard something that sounded like a scraping against the wall. He listened carefully, but it was gone.

Outside the wind had picked up, sending the rain against the window with a force that shook the glass in its frame. A car passed, its tires hissing over the wet street and its red taillights glowing in the darkness.

Greg thought he heard the noise again. His stomach tightened as he held himself still and listened intently. There weren't any more

---

2. **bodega** (boh DAY guh) *n.*: A small grocery store serving a Latino neighborhood.

Words to Know

impromptu (im PRAHMP too) *adj.*: Unscheduled, unplanned
ajar (uh JAR) *adj.*: Open
vaulted (VAWL tid) *v.*: Jumped over
tentatively (TEN tuh tiv lee) *adv.*: Hesitantly, with uncertainty
musty (MUS tee) *adj.*: Having a stale, moldy smell
intently (in TENT lee) *adv.*: Purposefully, carefully

---

1. **tenement** (TEN uh mint) *n.*: An old, run-down apartment house.

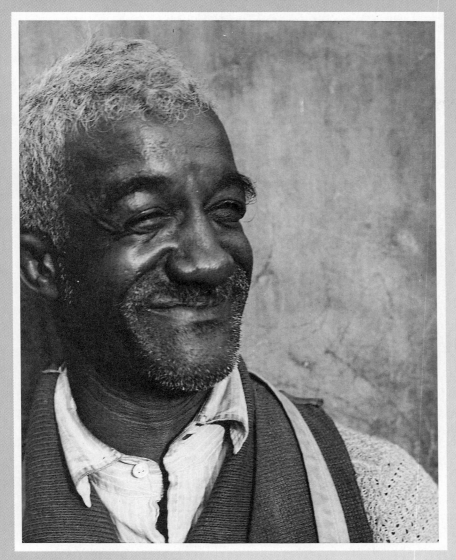

when he heard a voice behind him.

"Don't try nothin' 'cause I got a razor here sharp enough to cut a week into nine days!"

Greg, except for an involuntary tremor[3] in his knees, stood stock still. The voice was high and brittle, like dry twigs being broken, surely not one he had ever heard before.

📖 **Read Actively**

Predict what Greg will find in the tenement.

There was a shuffling sound as the person who had been speaking moved a step closer. Greg turned, holding his breath, his eyes straining to see in the dark room.

The upper part of the figure before him was still in darkness. The lower half was in the dim rectangle of light that fell unevenly from the window. There were two feet, in cracked, dirty shoes from which rose legs that were wrapped in rags.

"Who are you?" Greg hardly recognized his own voice.

"I'm Lemon Brown," came the answer. "Who're you?"

"Greg Ridley."

"What you doing here?" The figure shuffled forward again, and Greg took a small step backward.

"It's raining," Greg said.

"I can see that," the figure said.

scraping noises, but he was sure he had heard something in the darkness—something breathing!

He tried to figure out just where the breathing was coming from; he knew it was in the room with him. Slowly he stood, tensing. As he turned, a flash of lightning lit up the room, frightening him with its sudden brilliance. He saw nothing, just the overturned table, the pile of rags and an old newspaper on the floor. Could he have been imagining the sounds? He continued listening, but heard nothing and thought that it might have just been rats. Still, he thought, as soon as the rain let up he would leave. He went to the window and was about to look

---

3. involuntary (in VAH luhn teh ree) **tremor** (TREH muhr) *n.*: Automatic trembling or shaking.

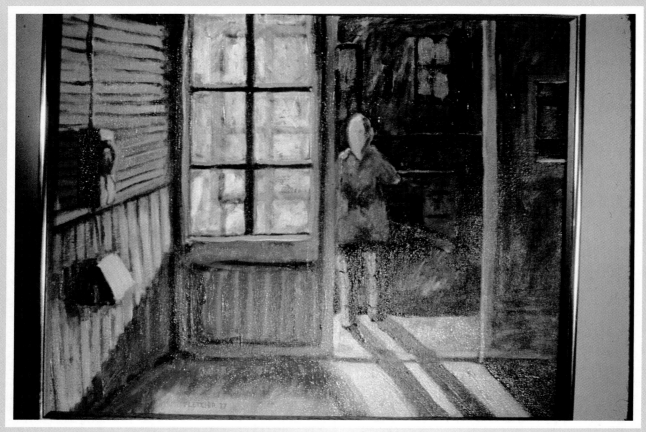

Morning at the Jackson–Ave Ferry Gilbert Fletcher, Courtesy of the artist

The person who called himself Lemon Brown peered forward, and Greg could see him clearly. He was an old man. His black, heavily wrinkled face was surrounded by a halo of crinkly white hair and whiskers that seemed to separate his head from the layers of dirty coats piled on his smallish frame. His pants were bagged to the knee, where they were met with rags that went down to the old shoes. The rags were held on with strings, and there was a rope around his middle. Greg relaxed. He had seen the man before, picking through the trash on the corner and pulling clothes out of a Salvation Army box. There was no sign of the razor that could "cut a week into nine days."

"What are you doing here?" Greg asked.

"This is where I'm staying," Lemon Brown said. "What you here for?"

"Told you it was raining out," Greg said, leaning against the back of the couch until he felt it give slightly.

"Ain't you got no home?"

"I got a home," Greg answered.

"You ain't one of them bad boys looking for my treasure, is you?" Lemon Brown cocked his head to one side and squinted one eye. "Because I told you I got me a razor."

"I'm not looking for your treasure," Greg answered, smiling. "*If* you have one."

"What you mean, *if* I have one," Lemon Brown said. "Every man got a treasure. You don't know that, you must be a fool!"

"Sure," Greg said as he sat on the sofa and put one leg over the back. "What do you have, gold coins?"

"Don't worry none about what I got," Lemon Brown said. "You know who I am?"

"You told me your name was orange or lemon or something like that."

"Lemon Brown," the old man said, pulling back his shoulders as he did so, "they used to call me Sweet Lemon Brown."

"Sweet Lemon?" Greg asked.

"Yessir. Sweet Lemon Brown. They used to say I sung the blues so sweet that if I sang at a funeral, the dead would commence to rocking with the beat. Used to travel all over Mississippi and as far as Monroe, Louisiana, and east on over to Macon, Georgia. You mean you ain't never heard of Sweet Lemon Brown?"

"Afraid not," Greg said. "What . . . what happened to you?"

"Hard times, boy. Hard times always after a poor man. One day I got tired, sat down to rest a spell and felt a tap on my shoulder. Hard times caught up with me."

"Sorry about that."

"What you doing here? How come you didn't go on home when the rain come? Rain don't bother you young folks none."

"Just didn't." Greg looked away.

"I used to have a knotty-headed boy just like you." Lemon Brown had half walked, half shuffled back to the corner and sat down against the wall. "Had them big eyes like you got, I used to call them moon eyes. Look into them moon eyes and see anything you want."

"How come you gave up singing the blues?" Greg asked.

"Didn't give it up," Lemon Brown said. "You don't give up the blues; they give you up. After a while you do good for yourself, and it ain't nothing but foolishness singing about how hard you got it. Ain't that right?"

"I guess so."

"What's that noise?" Lemon Brown asked, suddenly sitting upright.

Greg listened, and he heard a noise outside. He looked at Lemon Brown and saw the old man pointing toward the window.

Greg went to the window and saw three men, neighborhood thugs, on the stoop. One was carrying a length of pipe. Greg looked back toward Lemon Brown, who moved quietly across the room to the window. The old man looked out, then beckoned frantically for Greg to follow him. For a moment Greg couldn't move. Then he found himself following Lemon Brown into the hallway and up darkened stairs. Greg followed as closely as he

could. They reached the top of the stairs, and Greg felt Lemon Brown's hand first lying on his shoulder, then probing down his arm until he finally took Greg's hand into his own as they crouched in the darkness.

"They's bad men," Lemon Brown whispered. His breath was warm against Greg's skin.

"Hey! Rag man!" A voice called. "We know you in here. What you got up under them rags? You got any money?"

Silence.

"We don't want to have to come in and hurt you, old man, but we don't mind if we have to."

Lemon Brown squeezed Greg's hand in his own hard, gnarled fist.

There was a banging downstairs and a light as the men entered. They banged around noisily, calling for the rag man.

"We heard you talking about your treasure." The voice was slurred. "We just want to see it, that's all."

"You sure he's here?" One voice seemed to come from the room with the sofa.

"Yeah, he stays here every night."

"There's another room over there; I'm going to take a look. You got that flashlight?"

"Yeah, here, take the pipe too."

Greg opened his mouth to quiet the sound of his breath as he sucked it in uneasily. A beam of light hit the wall a few feet opposite him, then went out.

"Ain't nobody in that room," a voice said. "You think he gone or something?"

"I don't know," came the answer. "All I know is that I heard him talking about some kind of treasure. You know they found that shopping bag lady with that money in her bags."

"Yeah. You think he's upstairs?"

"Hey, old man, are you up there?"

Silence.

"Watch my back, I'm going up."

There was a footstep on the stairs, and the beam from the flashlight danced crazily along the peeling wallpaper. Greg held his breath. There was another step and a loud crashing noise as the man banged the pipe

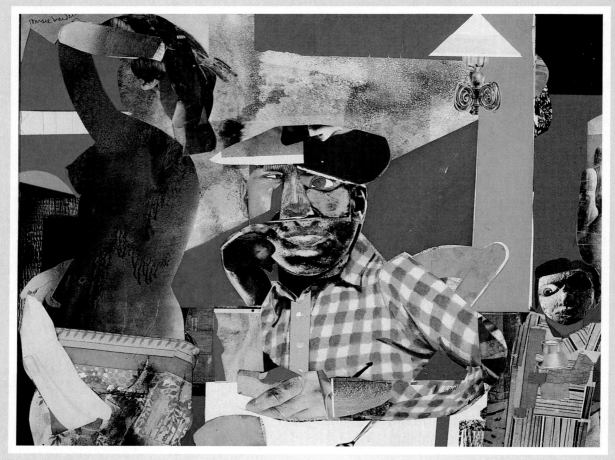

Sunrise, 1967 Romare Bearden, Courtesy Estate of Romare Bearden, ACA, Galleries New York and Munich

against the wooden banister.[4] Greg could feel his temples throb as the man slowly neared them. Greg thought about the pipe, wondering what he would do when the man reached them—what he *could* do.

Then Lemon Brown released his hand and moved toward the top of the stairs. Greg looked around and saw stairs going up to the next floor. He tried waving to Lemon Brown, hoping the old man would see him in the dim light and follow him to the next floor. Maybe, Greg thought, the man wouldn't follow them up there. Suddenly, though, Lemon Brown stood at the top of the stairs, both arms raised high above his head.

"There he is!" A voice cried from below.

"Throw down your money, old man, so I won't have to bash your head in!"

Lemon Brown didn't move. Greg felt him-self near panic. The steps came closer, and still Lemon Brown didn't move. He was an eerie sight, a bundle of rags standing at the top of the stairs, his shadow on the wall looming over him. Maybe, the thought came to Greg, the scene could be even eerier.

Greg wet his lips, put his hands to his mouth and tried to make a sound. Nothing came out. He swallowed hard, wet his lips once more and howled as evenly as he could.

"*What's that?*"

As Greg howled, the light moved away from Lemon Brown, but not before Greg saw him hurl his body down the stairs at the men who had come to take his treasure. There was a crashing noise, and then footsteps. A rush of warm air came in as the downstairs door opened, then there was only an ominous

📖 **Read Actively**

Ask yourself why Greg howls.

---

4. **banister** (BAN is tuhr) *n.*: Railing along a staircase.

silence.

Greg stood on the landing. He listened, and after a while there was another sound on the staircase.

"Mr. Brown?" he called.

"Yeah, it's me," came the answer. "I got their flashlight."

Greg exhaled in relief as Lemon Brown made his way slowly back up the stairs.

"You OK?"

"Few bumps and bruises," Lemon Brown said.

"I think I'd better be going," Greg said, his breath returning to normal. "You'd better leave, too, before they come back."

"They may hang around outside for a while," Lemon Brown said, "but they ain't getting their nerve up to come in here again. Not with crazy old rag men and howling spooks. Best you stay a while till the coast is clear. I'm heading out west tomorrow, out to east St. Louis."

"They were talking about treasures," Greg said. "You *really* have a treasure?"

📖 **Read Actively**

Predict what Lemon Brown's treasure will be.

"What I tell you? Didn't I tell you every man got a treasure?" Lemon Brown said. "You want to see mine?"

"If you want to show it to me," Greg shrugged.

"Let's look out the window first, see what them scoundrels be doing," Lemon Brown said.

They followed the oval beam of the flashlight into one of the rooms and looked out the window. They saw the men who had tried to take the treasure sitting on the curb near the corner. One of them had his pants leg up, looking at his knee.

"You sure you're not hurt?" Greg asked Lemon Brown.

"Nothing that ain't been hurt before," Lemon Brown said. "When you get as old as me all you say when something hurts is,

'Howdy, Mr. Pain, sees you back again.' Then when Mr. Pain see he can't worry you none, he go on mess with somebody else."

Greg smiled.

"Here, you hold this." Lemon Brown gave Greg the flashlight.

He sat on the floor near Greg and carefully untied the strings that held the rags on his right leg. When he took the rags away, Greg saw a piece of plastic. The old man carefully took off the plastic and unfolded it. He revealed some yellowed newspaper clippings and a battered harmonica.

"There it be," he said, nodding his head. "There it be."

Greg looked at the old man, saw the distant look in his eye, then turned to the clippings. They told of Sweet Lemon Brown, a blues singer and harmonica player who was appearing at different theaters in the South. One of the clippings said he had been the hit of the show, although not the headliner. All of the clippings were reviews of shows Lemon Brown had been in more than 50 years ago. Greg looked at the harmonica. It was dented badly on one side, with the reed holes on one end nearly closed.

"I used to travel around and make money for to feed my wife and Jesse—that's my boy's name. Used to feed them good, too. Then his mama died, and he stayed with his mama's sister. He growed up to be a man, and when the war come he saw fit to go off and fight in it. I didn't have nothing to give him except these things that told him who I was, and what he come from. If you know your pappy did something, you know you can do something too.

"Anyway, he went off to war, and I went off still playing and singing. 'Course by then I wasn't as much as I used to be, not without somebody to make it worth the while. You know what I mean?"

"Yeah," Greg nodded, not quite really knowing.

"I traveled around, and one time I come home, and there was this letter saying Jesse got killed in the war. Broke my heart, it truly did.

Words to Know

ominous (AHM uh nuhs) *adj.*: Threatening, frightening

"They sent back what he had with him over there, and what it was is this old mouth fiddle and these clippings. Him carrying it around with him like that told me it meant something to him. That was my treasure, and when I give it to him he treated it just like that, a treasure. Ain't that something?"

"Yeah, I guess so," Greg said.

"You *guess* so?" Lemon Brown's voice rose an octave as he started to put his treasure back into the plastic. "Well, you got to guess 'cause you sure don't know nothing. Don't know enough to get home when it's raining."

"I guess . . . I mean, you're right."

"You OK for a youngster," the old man said as he tied the strings around his leg, "better than those scalawags[5] what come here looking for my treasure. That's for sure."

"You really think that treasure of yours was worth fighting for?" Greg asked. "Against a pipe?"

"What else a man got 'cepting what he can pass on to his son, or his daughter, if she be his oldest?" Lemon Brown said. "For a big-headed boy you sure do ask the foolishest questions."

Lemon Brown got up after patting his rags in place and looked out the window again.

"Looks like they're gone. You get on out of here and get yourself home. I'll be watching from the window so you'll be all right."

📖 Read Actively

Make an **inference** about Lemon Brown. What does this comment tell you about him?

Lemon Brown went down the stairs behind Greg. When they reached the front door the old man looked out first, saw the street was clear and told Greg to scoot on home.

"You sure you'll be OK?" Greg asked.

"Now didn't I tell you I was going to east St. Louis in the morning?" Lemon Brown asked. "Don't that sound OK to you?"

"Sure it does," Greg said. "Sure it does. And you take care of that treasure of yours."

"That I'll do," Lemon said, the wrinkles

about his eyes suggesting a smile. "That I'll do."

The night had warmed and the rain had stopped, leaving puddles at the curbs. Greg didn't even want to think how late it was. He thought ahead of what his father would say and wondered if he should tell him about Lemon Brown. He thought about it until he reached his stoop, and decided against it. Lemon Brown would be OK, Greg thought, with his memories and his treasure.

Greg pushed the button over the bell marked Ridley, thought of the lecture he knew his father would give him, and smiled.

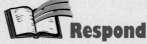

Respond

- Could meeting someone like Lemon Brown really change someone's way of thinking? Explain.
- With a partner, predict what happens to Greg in the weeks following this incident.

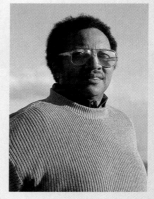

Walter Dean Myers
(1937–)
Q: How did Walter Dean Myers get his start as a writer?
A: A contest advertisement caught his attention. He wrote a story, sent it in, and won the $500 prize.
Q: What makes his writing special?
A: He is good at capturing the feel of the neighborhoods he describes.
Q: Why does he like to write for children and young adults?
A: He believes that young people are the future of the country. He enjoys getting mail from young readers who "see things in the books that [he] didn't even realize were there."

---

5. **scalawags** (SKAL uh wagz) *n.:* People who cause trouble; scoundrels.

Activities
MAKE MEANING

Explore Your Reading

Look Back (Recall)

1. List the facts you know about Greg.

Think It Over (Interpret)

2. What do you think Greg's first impression of Lemon Brown is?
3. What evidence shows that Greg's opinion of Lemon changes?
4. What lesson does Lemon Brown teach Greg?
5. Why do you think Greg smiles at the end of the story?

Go Beyond (Apply)

6. If you were to talk to someone younger about what matters most, what treasures would you share?

Develop Reading and Literary Skills

Appreciate Setting

Your diagram showed you the details that create a **setting**, or time and place, for this story. In some stories the setting is just a background for the action. In others, like this one, it plays a more special role, creating a mood and influencing the characters.

The abandoned building takes Greg out of his usual environment and causes him to look at things differently. Greg would not have met Lemon if he had not gone into the building, and he would not have stayed if it had not been raining. You could say, therefore, that the setting helps Greg to grow.

1. What mood or feeling does the setting create? Which details are especially important in creating this mood?
2. How does this mood make Greg pay more attention to Lemon?
3. Why does the danger of the setting make Lemon's treasure seem more valuable?
4. How would this story be different if Greg met Lemon Brown on a park bench on a sunny day?

Ideas for Writing

Imagine that you are involved in creating a stage production of "The Treasure of Lemon Brown."

Stage Set Design Write a proposal for the stage set for the new play. Identifying the key details of the setting, describe how the stage should look. You may want to suggest props, clothing, and colors to heighten the mood you want to create.

Credo Monologue Write a final speech that Greg will deliver to the audience as he thinks about the evening's events. Have him explain to the audience how his encounter with Lemon has influenced his personal beliefs.

Ideas for Projects

Space Capsule Create a set of the Earth's "treasures" that you would send into outer space. Have the collection show what matters most to our planet and its inhabitants. [Science Link]

Oral Report on Homelessness Lemon Brown is one of the homeless. Research the problem of homelessness in the United States by contacting organizations like the Salvation Army. Then present your findings to your classmates. [Social Studies Link]

Audio Presentation of the Blues Lemon Brown had been a Blues musician. Research this type of music, which grew out of African American culture. Record important songs and performers, and present your information in an audio history of the Blues. [Music Link; Social Studies Link]

How Am I Doing?

Answer these questions with a partner:

How did identifying details of setting help me better understand the message of this story?

Which example of my work will I put in my portfolio? Why?

What does thought add to an experience?

Reach Into Your Background

If experience is like uncooked food, thought is like the fire over which you can simmer it until it is ready to be eaten.

If experience is like a diamond, thought is like a hand that lets you hold the diamond in different ways to see all its facets.

These comparisons explore what it means to have an experience and then to think about it. With a partner, choose one of the sentences and put it in your own words. Then, use one or both of the following activities to continue the exploration:

*   With a partner, think of another comparison that describes having an experience and thinking about it.
*   Tell a partner about an experience that meant more to you after you thought about it.

Read Actively
Identify Elements of a Reflective Essay

Writers can think "out loud" about their experiences in a short work of nonfiction called a **reflective essay**. Such an essay usually has the following elements:

*   a writer telling about a personal experience, using the pronoun *I*
*   the writer's thoughts about the experience
*   a friendly, informal tone

By identifying these elements, you will be able to participate with a writer as he or she finds deeper meaning in an experience.

As you read "The Leader in the Mirror," jot down passages that reveal each of these elements in a chart like this one.

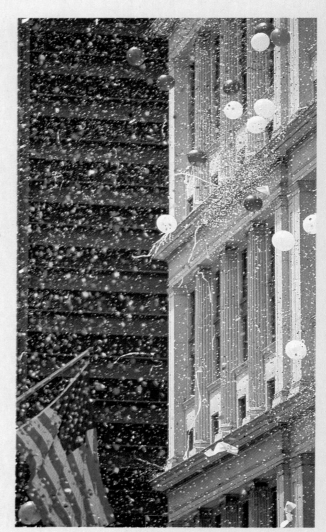

Personal experiences

Writer's thoughts

Friendly tone

The Leader in the Mirror

Pat Mora

Each year, the newspaper in my hometown of El Paso, Texas, honors the top five academic achievers from the local high schools at an annual banquet. Last year when I addressed the group, the room at the fancy hotel was full of proud students and their relatives. The aspirations of the students were like a dose of powerful vitamins, filling parents, educators and guests with energy.

I began by congratulating the family members and teachers for being steady beacons for those young people. In a society that undervalues families and educators, they had truly lived their commitments.

As I was planning the talk I would give to this group, I wondered how best to create an occasion for reflection. What could I say to the audience about the daily struggle to create a meaningful life?

I remembered planning parties for my children when they were young: the careful selection of party favors, the mementos for the guests to carry away.

Words to Know

aspirations (as puhr AY shunz) *n.*: Strong wishes, hopes, or ambitions

beacons (BEE kuhnz) *n.*: Shining examples

mementos (muh MEN tohs) *n.*: Souvenirs; keepsakes; objects to remind a person of something

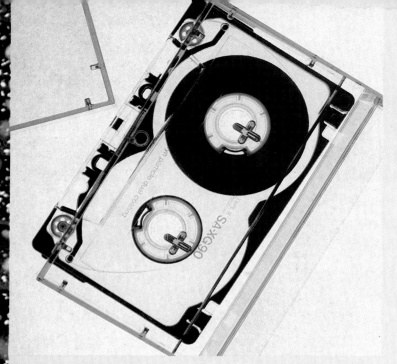

Since this banquet was to be a party of sorts, an academic celebration, I asked myself what favors I would choose for each place at the table.

I knew I would be very popular with the students if I could give them keys to a new red car or tickets to an island vacation. But I am a writer, not a millionaire. So I decided to give them imaginary gifts: Each student would receive confetti, a tape recorder, a photograph and a mirror—symbols and metaphors to take with them through life.

I hoped that most of the students were going to enroll in college. The confetti would be for their private celebrations, those solitary moments when they had passed a test that worried them, finished a difficult paper at 2 A.M., found a summer internship.[1] Sometimes, even when no one else is around, it's important to celebrate when we have struggled and succeeded—to sprinkle a little confetti on our own heads.

Why a tape recorder? I read them my poem "Immigrants."

> Immigrants
> wrap their babies in the American flag,
> feed them mashed hot dogs and apple pie,
> name them Bill and Daisy,
> buy them blonde dolls that blink blue
> eyes or a football and tiny cleats
> before the baby can even walk,
> speak to them in thick English,
>   hallo, babee, hallo,
> whisper in Spanish or Polish
> when the baby sleeps, whisper
> in a dark parent bed, that dark
> parent fear, "Will they like
> our boy, our girl, our fine american
> boy, our fine american girl?"

---

1. **internship** (IN tuhrn ship) *n.*: A job that helps young people learn about careers by training in specific businesses.

As a writer, I understand the value and necessity of knowing my past, of keeping that door open. My family stories are my catalyst[2] for creativity. All of us have people in our lives whose voices merit saving if we'll only take the time.

My own father was once a paper boy for the newspaper hosting the banquet. I might not have known that fact, nor his long history of hard work, had I not been listening to him with my tape recorder a few years ago. I did not want the students to wait as long as I had to begin preserving the rich inheritance of their family voices. The strength of their heritage would give them the courage to face the future.

My third gift was a photograph of the El Paso/Juarez border: the Chihuahua Desert, the Rio Grande,[3] a stern mountain, two sprawling border cities. Like our families, our geography is part of who we are.

When I was growing up on the U.S. side of that border, the society around me tried in subtle and not-so-subtle ways to convince me that my Mexican heritage was inferior to that of Anglo-Americans. I hope that today's educators on the border and throughout this nation are now committed to multiculturalism, to motivating the next generation to draw on their heritage as a resource for learning. The U.S. has been described as the first international country: Our varied cultures are our common wealth.

Borders—and if we're attentive, we realize we all live on borders, whether they are national or not—are sites of tension and sites for learning. Borders invite us to confront differences, inequities[4] and

---

2. **catalyst** (CAT uh list) *n.*: An inspiration.
3. **El Paso** (el PAH soh)/**Juarez** (WA rez) **border: the Chihuahua** (chee WAH wah) **Desert, the Rio Grande** (REE oh GRAHND eh): Border between El Paso, Texas, and Juarez, Mexico.
4. **inequities** (in EK wuht ees) *n.*: Unfairnesses; instances that reveal injustices.

Words to Know

preserving (pree ZUR ving) *v.*: Saving in a good condition; keeping
inheritance (in HER i tuhns) *n.*: A gift passed from one generation to the next
subtle (SUH tuhl) *adj.*: Sly; not open or direct

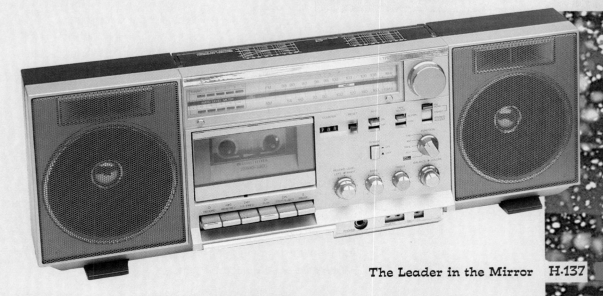

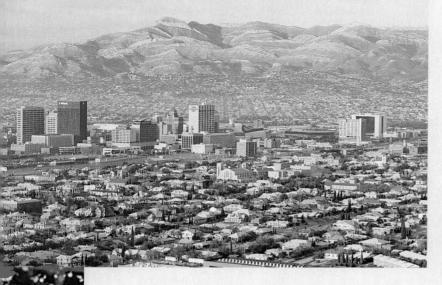

stereotypes. They invite us to work for multicultural cooperation and to celebrate multilingual richness.

The final gift of the evening, a mirror, was for serious gazing. I asked the students if they saw a leader when they looked into their mirrors. My guess is that too many of our young people do not see themselves as leaders because they don't look, dress or sound like the images of leaders presented to us. But leaders come in all colors, shapes and sizes. Some are talkative while others are quiet, but they all share a determination to contribute to the society of the future.

I urged the students to look often in their mirrors and to ask themselves these questions: "Am I satisfied with this world? If not, what will I do to improve it?" For if we are shaped by our surroundings, we in turn shape them. We deceive ourselves if we believe that we can live neutral lives.

One-third of this nation now traces its heritage to regions other than Western Europe. We will continue to squander our talent if our leaders—in politics, science, business, education and the arts—do not reflect our grand variety. I urged the students (and all of us) to ponder the strength of the mountains around us, to rise to the challenges.

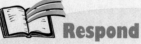 **Respond**

- In what areas can you be a leader?
- With a partner, discuss imaginary gifts that you might give friends or family.

Words to Know

squander (SKWAHN duhr) *v.*: Waste; spend foolishly
ponder (PAHN duhr) *v.*: Think deeply about; consider carefully

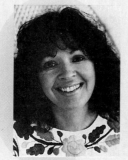

PAT MORA

Q: Where was Pat Mora raised?
A: She grew up in El Paso, Texas, on the United States/Mexico border.
Q: How have borders been important in her own writing?
A: In this essay, Mora describes the importance of borders in her own life. She even named a volume of her poetry *Borders*.
Q: What does Mora write about?
A: Her award-winning short stories and poems are about her experience as a Mexican American.

MAKE MEANING

Explore Your Reading

Look Back (Recall)

1. What explanation does Mora give for each of the gifts she discusses?

Think It Over (Interpret)

2. Why did the writer read the poem "Immigrants" to her audience?
3. How are "[our] varied cultures . . . our common wealth"?
4. Which of Mora's imaginary gifts is the most valuable? In answering, consider how these gifts might help you.

Go Beyond (Apply)

5. Which symbolic gifts do you take with you through life? Explain.

Develop Reading and Literary Skills

Analyze a Reflective Essay

Your chart showed you how Mora uses this **reflective essay** as a way of thinking further about the experience of planning and giving a speech.

The essay also offers her an opportunity to share her experience, and her thoughts about it, with a new audience of readers. The speech itself only reached a limited number of listeners. Through this essay, however, Mora can give her symbolic gifts to anyone who reads her words.

In addition, those who heard her speech could not know how she created it. Readers of the essay can relive the experience of planning the speech and making discoveries that went into it.

1. Find an example of Mora's informal, conversational style and show how it helps her to reach out to readers.
2. Identify a passage in which Mora thinks further about her experience. Explain how her thoughts add to the experience.

3. In your own words, summarize what you think she learned from giving the speech and reflecting on it in the essay.

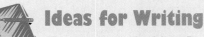

Ideas for Writing

"The Leader in the Mirror" may encourage you to think about what it takes to be a leader. It might even inspire you to exercise leadership.

Graduation Speech Write a graduation speech that you might deliver to your classmates. Like Mora, give listeners symbolic gifts that will help them in their lives.

How-to Manual Create a manual that shows how to be a leader. Consider writing sections on leadership in sports, student government, schoolwork, and other areas of school life.

Ideas for Projects

Leadership Training Research opportunities for leadership training in your community. You might start by checking at the library or a community center. Report your findings to the class. [Social Studies Link]

Dance Create a dance that demonstrates the qualities of a good leader. You can compose your own music or use something already recorded. You might even want to have a narrator. Perform your dance for your classmates. [Music Link]

How Am I Doing?

Take a moment to write responses to these questions:

How did identifying the elements of a reflective essay help me understand this selection? How can I apply what I learned to other reading?

What does this article say to me about deciding what matters most?

How do you make your decisions?

Reach Into Your Background

How you make a decision may depend on the importance of *what* you're deciding. "Which cleanser?" is an easier decision than "Which college?" You may have noticed, however, that people have styles of decision-making. Some are more willing to make decisions based on the flip of a coin or the flip of a feeling. Others may debate the pros and cons of which snack to buy.

Think further about decisions by deciding to do one or both of these activities:

- Analyze your own style of decision-making. Are you quick or slow? Are you ruled by thoughts, feelings, or both?
- In a group, role-play a humorous situation in which a slow, thoughtful decision-maker and a quick, breezy one try to choose a movie they'll see.

Read Actively

Recognize Forms in Poetry

Poets make decisions too. For example, they choose a **poetic form**, or pattern, for their work. If they write in free verse, they'll use lines of different lengths and varied patterns of stressed syllables. If they write more formal poems, they'll use regular patterns of stressed syllables and predictable rhymes, the like-sounding words at the ends of lines. By recognizing poetic forms, you'll understand the choices poets make. You'll also be able to think about the reasons for these stylistic choices.

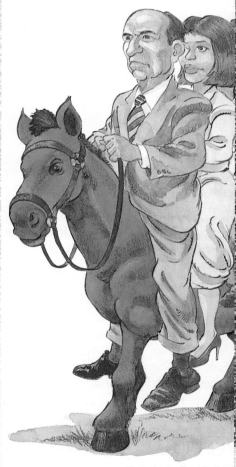

Illustration by Steve Haefele

As you read these poems, recognize their forms by jotting down examples of regular rhythms and rhymes or of free verse. If you're unsure of the rhythm, read the line slowly to yourself and emphasize the stressed syllables.

An Easy Decision

Kenneth Patchen

I had finished my dinner
Gone for a walk
It was fine
Out and I started whistling

5   It wasn't long before

I met a
Man and his wife riding on
A pony with seven
Kids running along beside them

10   I said hello and

Went on
Pretty soon I met another
Couple
This time with nineteen
15   Kids and all of them
Riding on
A big smiling hippopotamus

I invited them home

📖 **Read Actively**
Make an **inference**. What does his whistling tell you about the speaker?

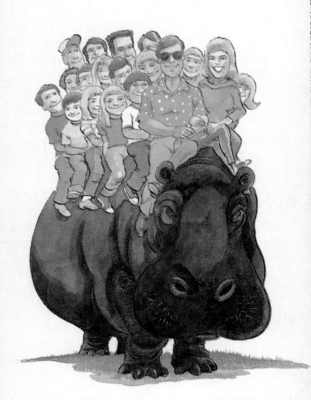

Illustration by Steve Haefele

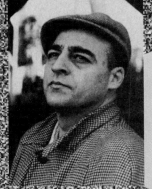

Although **Kenneth Patchen** (1911–1972) had a painful spinal disease for most of his life, he wrote or painted for at least twenty minutes every day from the time he was twelve. He said, "I have never let my pain stop my work, because the pain is less important."

Stopping by Woods on a Snowy Evening

Robert Frost

Whose woods these are I think I know.
His house is in the village, though;
He will not see me stopping here
To watch his woods fill up with snow.

5   My little horse must think it queer
To stop without a farmhouse near
Between the woods and frozen lake
The darkest evening of the year.

He gives his harness bells a shake
10   To ask if there is some mistake.
The only other sound's the sweep
Of easy wind and downy flake.

The woods are lovely, dark, and deep,
But I have promises to keep,
15   And miles to go before I sleep,
And miles to go before I sleep.

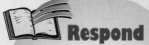

Read Actively

Visualize this winter scene.

Respond
- What choices, large or small, have you made recently?
- Choose one of these poems and read it aloud to a partner.

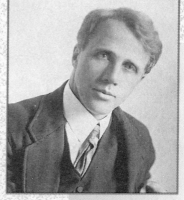

Many of the poems of **Robert Frost** (1874–1963), like "Stopping by Woods," are set in New England. They describe with precision and care the look of the region's landscape and the concerns of its people. However, they also deal with the universal themes of loneliness, love, and fear.

If you read more of Frost's poetry, you will see that he was a master craftsman, too. Each of his poems is as well made as a good New England ax handle.

Activities
MAKE MEANING

 Explore Your Reading

Look Back (Recall)

1. Describe what happens in each poem.

Think It Over (Interpret)

2. Why was Kenneth Patchen's decision an easy one to make?
3. Why do you think Frost stops by himself in such a lonely spot?
4. What kinds of "promises" make Frost continue on his way?

Go Beyond (Apply)

5. How does each of these poems answer the question "What matters most?"

 Develop Reading and Literary Skills

Appreciate Poetic Forms

You've seen the **poetic forms**, or patterns, each of these poets chose for his work. Patchen wrote in **free verse**, with lines of varying lengths and different rhythms ("It was FINE / OUT and I STARted WHIStling"). Frost, however, wrote in more formal verse, with regular rhythms and rhymes ("He GIVES his HARness BELLS a SHAKE / To ASK if THERE is SOME misTAKE").

Each poet has chosen a form that is best suited to the mood and message he wants to convey. For example, the lack of regular rhyme and rhythm in Patchen's poem adds to its humor. You don't know how long or short the next line will be, or what surprising and funny image it will contain.

1. Find another passage showing the free verse of Patchen's poem and one showing the regular forms of Frost's poem. Explain your choices.
2. Why are predictable rhythms and rhymes more suited to the mood of Frost's poem?

Ideas for Writing

Both of these poets recognize that we make choices all the time.

Limerick Some choices that you've made or observed have probably had humorous results. Write a limerick about one of these choices. Here's an example of the form:

> A flea and a fly in a flue
> Were caught, so what could they do?
> Said the fly, "Let us flee."
> "Let us fly," said the flea.
> So they flew through a flaw in the flue.

Interpretation Choose a character from life, a movie, or a television show and explain a choice he or she made. Describe the person's options, the final decision, and the reasons for it.

Ideas for Projects

Consumer Report People constantly make decisions about what to buy. Choose an item that is popular among your classmates. Then, research several brands of the product, comparing quality, price, and other important factors. Present your findings in a chart or graph that will help classmates make a purchasing decision. [Math Link]

Career Panel Careers also involve decisions. Invite experts from different fields to come to class and discuss how to choose a career. Ask them to answer questions that you have prepared. [Social Studies Link; Science Link; Math Link; Art Link]

How Am I Doing?

Take a moment to discuss these questions with a partner:

How did recognizing forms of poetry help me understand these poems better? How can I apply what I have learned to other poems?

Which piece of work would I like to save in my portfolio?

What job opportunities did teenagers have in medieval times?

Reach Into Your Background

WANTED: Teenaged apprentice to a famous painter.
LIVING QUARTERS: Behind the workshop, with the other apprentices.
DUTIES: Make charcoal sticks for drawing; prepare parchment; bring breakfast for the apprentices each morning.
OPPORTUNITY: Learn the art of painting from a master.

If you lived in Europe around the year 1200, you may have seen signs like this. Look ahead at the pictures in this selection and see the work of the man who took this position. Then think more about job opportunities in the Middle Ages by doing one or both of these:

- In a group, brainstorm to list the questions you would like to ask a medieval teenager about his or her life.
- With a partner, role-play a job interview based on the wanted notice that appears above.

Read Actively
Connect Literature to Social Studies

Sometimes what you've learned in social studies will help you understand a work of literature. For example, you've probably studied the Middle Ages and learned about serfs who farmed the land and knights who defended their lords' castles. When reading true or fictional stories about the Middle Ages, you'll enjoy them more if you connect them to what you already know about this time.

As you read this historical biography, or life of a famous person from the past, jot down what you know and learn by filling in a chart like this one:

The Life of a Medieval Painter		
What I Know	What I Want to Know	What I've Learned

The Boy Who Drew Sheep

Anne Rockwell

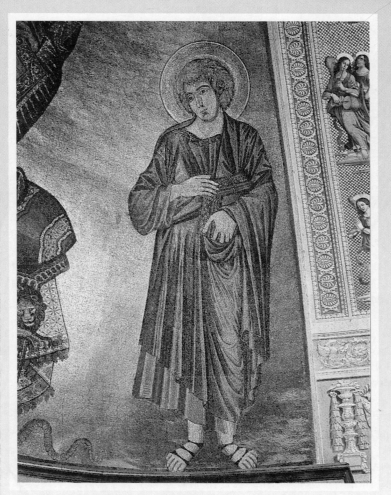

St. John the Evangelist, Apse Mosaic, Pisa Duomo
Cimabue, Art Resource, New York

M ore than seven hundred years ago, in a valley in Italy, there lived a farmer named Bondone. He had a wife and a house, some pigs, a few cows, fig and olive trees, many, many woolly sheep, and a son to help him on the farm. The boy was named Giotto.[1] When he was nine years old, his father entrusted the flock of sheep to him. Each morning, before the sun was up, Giotto and his dog led the sheep up into the hills where they nibbled all day at the meadow grass; and in the evening, when the moon rose, he led them safely home again.

Alone as he was, with no playmates or companions but his dog and sheep, Giotto began to pass the long days by scratching pictures with a sharp pebble on the large stones that jutted up here and there in the meadow. First he drew the things that came into his head, but after a while he decided to draw something that he had actually seen. And so he began to make a picture of one of his sheep. He worked and worked, but the drawing never seemed quite right. So when he finished one he would begin another. The time passed quickly this way, and wherever he wandered with his flock, the rocks were scratched with pictures of sheep: old and solemn rams, gentle ewes, and curly baby lambs.

One day a group of gentlemen on horseback came riding up into the hills where Giotto herded his flock. Both men and horses were dressed in the finest and shiniest silk and leather. Each gentleman carried a hawk on his wrist, and each hawk wore a little leather mask on his face. The men

---

1. Giotto (JAH toh)

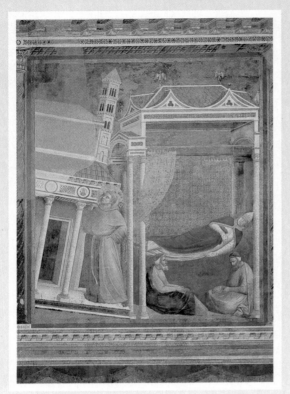

*(The Dream of Pope Innocent III) Vita di S. Francesco -
Il sogno di Innocenzo III* Giotto, Art Resource, New York

were hunting. But Giotto did not notice them, so busy was he with his newest drawing. Not far from where he sat, a little spring of fresh, cold water gushed up between two rocks. One of the gentlemen rode over all alone, and he and his horse drank from the cool water. While he was at the spring, he noticed the boy. So he walked quietly over and looked at the drawing.

Giotto must have been surprised to see the well-dressed stranger, for few people came into his hills. The gentleman introduced himself as Cimabue,[2] a citizen of the city of Florence.[3] He congratulated Giotto on his fine drawing and said that he too was an artist. He painted pictures on the walls of the churches of Florence. The man looked again at Giotto's drawing and then offered to teach Giotto all of the many things he knew about picture painting. Giotto would have to come and work for him in his

---

2. **Cimabue** (chee mah BOO eh)
3. **Florence** (FLAHR uhns): The Italian city often called the birthplace of the Renaissance since many of the period's great artists lived or worked there.

workshop, of course, if this were to happen. Giotto was surprised by this, for where he lived most men were farmers and shepherds, as their fathers had been and their sons would be, and there were no artists.

That evening, when the boy led the sheep back to the valley, Cimabue went with him. For a long time he spoke with Giotto's mother and father. He told them that of all the boys who had ever worked in his workshop (and there were many), none could draw so well, without any lessons, as their son Giotto.

The farmer Bondone was a practical man. He didn't want his son to waste his time in foolishness. But as he looked at the stranger's elegant clothes, which must have cost a great deal of money, he began to think that perhaps the stranger was right: Giotto should go and learn to paint pictures. Perhaps he too would grow rich. And so, before the family went to bed that night, it was settled. Giotto would go to Florence and become an apprentice in Cimabue's workshop.

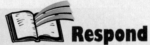

Respond

How do you think Giotto feels when he learns that he is going to Florence?

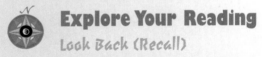

Explore Your Reading

Look Back (Recall)

1. How does Giotto first show his talent as an artist?

Think It Over (Interpret)

2. What kind of a man is Cimabue?

2

Early next morning Giotto, instead of heading for the hills with his sheep, said good-bye to them and to his dog and to his mother and father. He climbed up in back of Cimabue on the painter's high-stepping horse, and the two of them set off toward Florence.

Many hours later they reached the gates of the city. Tall towers bristled proudly against

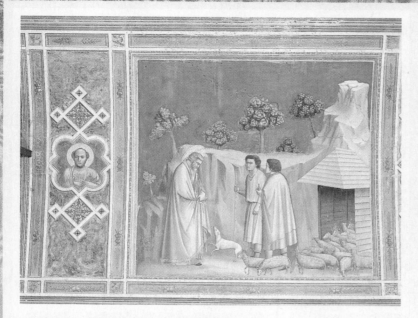

(Joachim Among the Shepherds) Giovacchino tra i pastori
Giotto, Art Resource, New York

the sky, and inside the strong walls were more people together than Giotto had seen in his whole life. Knights in armor rode through the busy streets; well-dressed merchants talked together of business; market stalls were filled to overflowing with sweet figs and melons and other good things from the hills.

On every corner, or so it seemed, women sat chatting and spinning wool into long skeins.[4] Iron hooks projected from nearly all of the houses in Florence. Across these iron hooks lay cross-pieces of wood. And from these wooden cross-pieces hung great skeins of purple, crimson, gold, and deep blue wool, drying in the air. For the city of Florence was rich from wool, wool from the sheep that shepherds such as Giotto had raised in the hills. This good wool of Florence was sold to the world and the city's wool merchants were rich and proud.

The city was grand and glorious. Its churches were filled with pictures painted by artists such as Cimabue, artists all other cities in the world would have liked to have. The pictures covered the plaster walls of churches or hung from strong wooden panels. They gleamed with brilliant red and blue and paper-thin coatings of real gold, bright as the sun.

Cimabue took Giotto to the workshop, which stood on one of Florence's narrow, busy streets. There the boy was introduced to the other apprentices. Some of them were boys nearly as young as Giotto; others were almost men; and one or two were grown men without workshops of their own. They managed the workshop of Cimabue. The apprentices lived together behind the workshop. Giotto was welcomed as one of them, and his training began.

First he learned to make charcoal sticks for drawing. He cut up several willow switches into lengths just a little longer than his longest finger. Then he carefully sharpened each end to a point with his knife. Next he tied all of the willow sticks into several neat bundles. These bundles went into an earthenware casserole, with a cover. When the bundles were in, he sealed the cover of the casserole tight shut with a shaped piece of clay, so the inside was airtight. Last of all, he carefully carried the pot to the baker's shop. He gave it to the baker, who placed it at the entrance of one of the great ovens that he was lighting that night for the baking of fine loaves of bread early in the morning. And that night, all night long, the casserole sat in the baker's oven, while the boy slept and dreamed that the charcoal sticks would turn out well. For if the fire was too hot, or the willow bundles improperly packed, the charcoal would be too burnt, and it would crumble when it was put to paper or parchment. Then the boy who made it might be whipped. But if he was lucky and had done

---

4. **skeins** (SKAYNZ) *n.*: Loose thick coils.

Words to Know

parchment (PARCH muhnt) *n.*: The skin of a sheep or goat that has been prepared so that it can be written or painted on

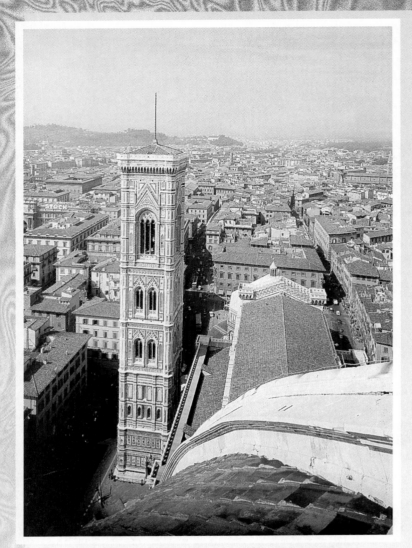

The Campanile: Giotto's bell tower in Florence's Piazza del Duomo

burned them in the fire until the ashes were white and soft. These ashes were ground on a smooth stone slab until they were even softer. Then, with a furry rabbit's foot, he dusted the powder back and forth, back and forth across the dried skin until it was velvet smooth and ready to take the lines made by charcoal, or if more delicate work was wanted, by a little piece of tarnished silver wire from the goldsmith's workshop.

And all the time he was learning these things, Giotto, in the little time he had left for himself, drew pictures . . . just as he had while he tended his father's sheep in the high hills.

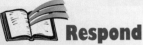

Respond

What pictures do you think Giotto draws in his spare time?

 ## Explore Your Reading

Look Back (Recall)

1. What sights in Florence are new to Giotto?

Go Beyond (Apply)

2. Is there a system of apprenticeship today? Explain.

his work well, the sticks would be hard and black, and there would be charcoal for drawing for many weeks, and praise for him, too. When Giotto brought his first charcoal back to the workshop, he *was* lucky, for the sticks were perfect, black and sharp and crisp. He also brought breakfast . . . the first loaves of the morning, warm and round and crusty.

He learned to prepare parchment for drawing. From the leather tanner, pieces of skin from a very young calf were bought. These he washed, nailed to a wooden stretcher, and dried in the sunshine. Then, he picked up the chicken bones from under the dining table at night, where the apprentices threw them, and

3

Sometimes the other apprentices told him stories of the glory that came to a painter as skilled and admired as their master. Once Cimabue had received a commission to paint a picture of the Virgin Mary. She was to be surrounded by angels, and she would sit against a sky of gold. The picture would hang in a church in Florence in a spot where all would see it, including the visiting foreign kings and princes who came to Florence. It was springtime when Cimabue began the painting. One day the breezes blew so soft and pleasant, and the air smelled so sweetly of violets, that

Cimabue moved his easel outdoors to his garden to paint. A neighbor, watching from a window, saw the picture and passed the word to a friend that it was more beautiful than anyone could possibly imagine. Word spread through the city, and next morning, when Cimabue came out to paint, many many people were already peeping over his garden wall to watch him while he worked. Even the king of France, who happened to be passing through Florence, joined the citizens as they stood and watched.

"How beautiful!" everyone said, as Cimabue painted in an apple-pink cheek.

"How glorious!" they said, as he burnished[5] the gold-leaf background with the smooth tooth of an ox, until the gold was dark and shining.

When the painting was done, the citizens nearly wept with joy at the sight of it; and they decided that a picture as special as this one needed as special a journey as possible to the church where it was to hang. And so on the day the painting made its journey from the workshop to the church, it was accompanied by a grand parade of fifers,[6] tambour drummers and trumpeters—and by everyone in the city, or so it seemed. Every apprentice hoped that such fame would one day come to him. Every young painter hoped that one day he would make pictures as fine as the pictures of Cimabue.

But for Giotto it was enough for now to draw and to hope that one day his master would say, "Here Giotto, paint in the face of this angel—the one in the far-left corner." Giotto worked, and he drew, and he lived the life of an apprentice.

---

5. burnished (BER nisht) *v.*: Polished.
6. fifers (FĪ fuhrs): Musicians playing small flutes.

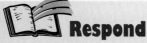

Respond

Would you have liked to live in medieval Florence? Why or why not?

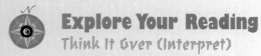

Explore Your Reading

Think It Over (Interpret)

1. Describe how an apprentice might advance.

Go Beyond (Apply)

2. In what ways was the medieval world smaller than ours?

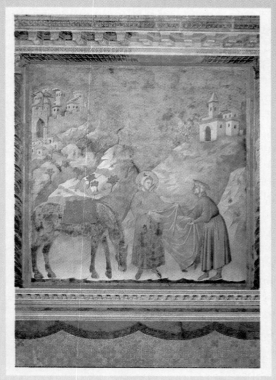

(Life of St. Francis: St. Francis Giving His Cloak to the Poor)
Storie di S. Francesco: il dono del mantello
Giotto, Art Resource, New York

4

At the time Giotto lived, in the city of Florence as in other cities, only the boys of the rich went to school. All other boys learned a trade. They were apprenticed to master craftsmen, who provided food, clothing and shelter, as well as learning. In return the boys worked for the master.

In Florence there was a strange custom that Giotto must have enjoyed. Each day when noontime came, all of the apprentices from all of the trades in the city left their workshops and ran to the marketplace for lunch. There they feasted on sausages and fresh figs, and drank cool sweet lemonade from the lemon vendor's stall faster than the poor man could squeeze it. But sometimes fights broke out between apprentices: the wooldyers fought with the painters; the carpenters fought with the apothecaries;[7] the goldsmiths fought with the

---

7. apothecaries (uh PAHTH uh ker eez) *n.*: Pharmacists; druggists.

sculptors; for each trade thought its own the best. At times like that the market ran wild, and geese ran cackling shrilly underfoot; stall-keepers shouted vainly to the boys to stop while onions and lemons turned to weapons and went flying through the air. But suddenly the market bell would clang out loudly over the shouting and swearing, and the apprentices would return to work, always promising to finish the fight the next day. As they left, the unfortunate stall-keepers would sigh and swear and once more pile their goods neat and high.

Back at the workshop, Giotto and his fellow apprentices would dig into their work, having had their fling for the day. In Cimabue's workshop the apprentices were treated kindly. Although they worked hard, they ate well and slept in clean and comfortable beds.

But there were some painters who treated their apprentices badly and made them work too hard. One old painter, a stingy man, had but one apprentice, who was as lazy as his master was stingy. Each morning, in the cold darkness before dawn, the master woke the apprentice and set him hard at work grinding colors, preparing panels of wood and making brushes; then when day came the master could paint angels, although, to tell the truth, his angels were not beautiful. The lazy apprentice so hated waking up while it was still dark and shivery that he made up his mind to put a stop to it. Since he was not only lazy but an untidy housekeeper, in all corners of the workshop and under every piece of furniture, dust lay thick. Little creepy beetles lived in the dust. And one night while his master slept, the apprentice caught many, many of these little

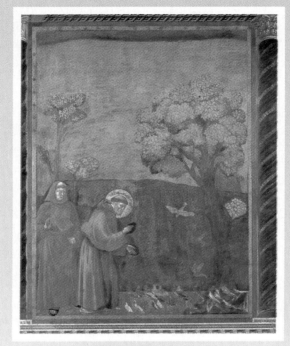

St. Francis preaching to the birds
Giotto, Art Resource, New York

beetles. With a tiny dripping of wax, he fastened a very small candle to each beetle's back. Then, after lighting each candle, he set the beetle army loose in his master's bedroom and hid in the hall. As the beetles slowly proceeded across the floor, like a long, silent, flaming dragon, the old painter wakened and shouted and screamed in terror, while the apprentice sat outside giggling silently. When morning came, the painter, in a trembling voice, told the apprentice of the terrible thing that had happened in the night.

"I am sure," he said, "that those were demons come to get me. They are very angry because I have been painting so many angels, for angels are good and demons are bad! But the night belongs to strange monsters! Let us leave it to them; from now on we work no more until the sun, which chases away demons, is fully up in the morning."

And so it was that the lazy apprentice could sleep late in the morning. Indeed in all the workshops of Florence, everyone heard of the flaming demons and took heed; and from that time on, work was done only in daylight hours.

That did not stop apprentices from playing other tricks, however. Giotto, too, invented some. He was now allowed to paint small portions of the master's canvases himself. One day he painted a tiny fly on the nose of a figure on a panel. He giggled as his master tried unsuccessfully to brush it off, for he thought it was real. And although Cimabue would not admit it, the boy's joke also gave him pleasure, for it showed that the young shepherd from the hills was learning his trade remarkably well.

But there was much more to being a painter than painting a fly to fool the eye. Giotto had to make brushes, delicate brushes of ermine[8] tails for small and precise work, and hard strong bristle brushes made from the back hairs of a white pig for more general work. He learned to grind the priceless chunks of color that he had gotten from the apothecary shop. He would grind and grind until they seemed to be as fine as dust; but then, when he showed them to his master, they would still be too coarse.

"Grind them," the master would say, "until you are sure you have ground them enough, and then grind them some more."

And so he would grind them again, and then again. But at last they would be ready and he would place them in neat little pots. There were all of the colors. Some were made of ground-up stones or earth, and some were products of the mysterious arts of the alchemist.[9] Some behaved strangely when mixed with other colors and therefore had to be used pure. There were still others that were highly poisonous. All of the rules for the use of all of the colors had to be learned before a painter could be sure that his pictures would not turn black in a short time.

Even worse, a painter who was careless of the way he handled some of the paint could develop symptoms of poisoning. He must not lick his brushes to make a point for delicate work. He must not inhale too much of the finely ground colored dust before it was mixed with water or oil or egg white to make it ready to spread on a picture.

The craft of a painter was filled with things that seemed magical and mysterious to those who had not learned the craft. And the images that grew on walls and panels, with blue made of precious ground lapis lazuli and reds of rare and rich cinnabar from Spain, and bright gold gleaming, seemed magical and mysterious to those who looked at them. But Giotto was now a part of those mysteries. He was becoming a painter.

---

8. **ermine** (UR muhn) *adj.*: From the northern European weasel.

9. **alchemist** (AL kuh mist) *n.*: Someone who practiced alchemy, a medieval form of chemistry. Alchemists tried to turn common metals into gold.

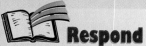

Respond

Why do you think the apprentices got into fights at lunchtime?

Explore Your Reading
Think It Over (Interpret)

1. In what way is a craft a "mystery"?

Go Beyond (Apply)

2. What does this chapter tell you about the relationship between masters and apprentices?

5

The years passed, and the boy Giotto grew up. Wherever he went he looked at people and at the world around him. He noticed the way people stood and moved in the busy marketplace, and he noticed the way they looked when they laughed or cried. He watched the way the long drapery of their clothing fell in rich folds to the ground when they walked or gestured. And always he drew what he saw, as he had done up in the hills. But now it was different, for he had learned so many things that he could draw well whatever he wished. He had mastered all of the many skills he needed to be a painter with a workshop of his own. Indeed, there were many people who said that he surpassed his master, the most famous painter in the land.

Giotto was soon called upon by the neighboring town of Assisi to paint some pictures for them.

Nearly one hundred years earlier a man called Francis had been born in Assisi. He was the son of a rich merchant, but he gave up all of his money and fine clothes and called himself, "the Little Poor Man." As a beggar, he wandered throughout Italy doing good things. Not only did he love people, but he loved the sun

Words to Know

surpassed (ser PAST) *v.*: Was better than; went beyond a limit

and moon as if they were his brother and sister, and he loved all of the birds and creatures of the earth. He even seemed able to speak to wild animals in their own language. He wrote poems and songs in praise of the wild things of the earth. These were written in the language

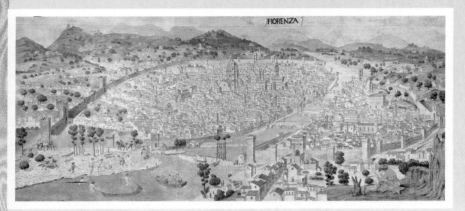

Map of Florence, Italy, in 1480
Stefano Buonsignori Scala/Art Resource, New York

the people around him spoke every day, instead of the Latin of learned poets. He wanted to teach people to live together more happily, and at the same time he wanted to teach them to share the earth with the birds and flowers, wild wolves, and fire and water and cold winter wind. After he died he became known as Saint Francis, and his native town wished to honor him by building a church dedicated to him. Giotto was asked to decorate the church with murals, telling stories from the life of Saint Francis. And so Giotto journeyed to Assisi to begin the work.

First, carpenters constructed a strong wooden scaffolding where he could stand with his assistants to reach the high walls where they would make the paintings. Next the bare stone walls were covered with a rough coat of plaster. Upon this plaster Giotto drew with charcoal, carefully copying and enlarging a small picture he had drawn previously on paper. Then he went over the charcoal with a little brush and brown paint, until the whole picture could easily be seen on the plaster. When he was ready to begin the finished painting, he mixed a small amount of fine smooth plaster and covered with it just enough of the wall with the picture drawn on for one day's

work. While the plaster was still wet, although set, he painted the parts of the picture that were in that area, using his dry colors mixed with water. The next day he again plastered a small area and painted it, generally the section adjoining the section he had finished the day before. Day after day he worked in this way. Many, many months passed, or perhaps longer, before the murals were done.

Then at last, there they stood, row after row of grand and bright paintings. Scenes from the life of Saint Francis covered the walls like pages from an enormous picture book for people to see, many of whom could neither read nor write.

These paintings were not like any that people had seen before. The pictures people of Giotto's time knew were stiff and unreal, painted in a way handed down from master to apprentice for hundreds of years. They looked more like other pictures than they looked like real life. But Giotto, like Saint Francis, had looked at the world around him and had seen that it was beautiful. He painted trees and animals, prickly plants and meadow flowers, strong boulders and tall city walls. But what was most unusual was the way he painted people. He filled many spaces with people, people who moved and smiled and cried and gestured as real people do, but who were larger than life. People loved what they saw in Giotto's pictures, but when they looked at him, they laughed, for

Words to Know

murals (MYOO ruhlz) *n.* : Images painted directly on walls

scaffolding (SKAF uhl ding) *n.*: A framework put up to support workers while they are building, repairing or painting something

adjoining (uh JOY ning) *adj.*: Next to; near

forfeit (FOR fit) *v.*: Give up or lose something

commissioned (kuh MISH und) *v.*: Hired

they said he was as small and ugly as his pictures were large and beautiful.

From city to city Giotto went, climbing scaffoldings and covering wall after wall with pictures. One day after painting many pictures in many cities, he was walking down a narrow alley in Florence, chatting with a friend. He did not notice a runaway pig escaping from the butcher's stall in the marketplace. Squealing shrilly, the pig took one look at Giotto, headed straight toward him and darted between the painter's legs, tripping him up, head over heels. As he pulled himself up and brushed the dirt from his clothes, Giotto laughed and said, "That pig must have known I am the painter who has used so many of his brothers' back bristles for brushes. I have made a great deal of money with my pig-bristle brushes, but I have never given a pig even a bowl of leftovers. Now, at last, I have paid my debt to pigs!"

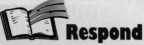 **Respond**

Did you picture Giotto as "small and ugly"? Why or why not?

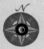 **Explore Your Reading**

Look Back (Recall)

1. How are Giotto's paintings different from those done by earlier artists?

Think It Over (Interpret)

2. Why is Giotto a good choice to paint the life of St. Francis?

6

In the city of Padua[10] there had lived a man called Scrovegni. He was a wicked man who loaned money to people and then charged such high rates of interest that they could not pay, and sometimes had to forfeit land or goods instead. When he died, he was very rich, but he was hated, by all who had heard of him, for his greed and cruelty. His son decided to use his father's great wealth to build a fine church for

_____
10. Padua (PAD yoo uh): The oldest city in Northern Italy.

the city, so that his father would be remembered for this instead of for his crimes. The son commissioned Giotto, who was by then more famous than Cimabue or any painter had ever been, to cover the walls of the new church with scenes from the life of Jesus. Some say that Giotto even helped the stonemasons plan the church, to make certain that he had plenty of wall space for his pictures. The son of the thief had planned well, for today people come from all over the world to look at Giotto's pictures, and the Scrovegni family is still remembered for the beautiful paintings in the chapel that bears its name.

One day a messenger came to Giotto from faraway Avignon,[11] in France. This was the city where the Pope lived at that time. The messenger had been sent to many artists in Italy, all of the best painters, to ask them to submit a painting for a contest. The prize would be a chance to do some well-paid work in Avignon. All of the artists the messenger approached worked very hard on their samples for the contest. But when the messenger asked Giotto for his picture, Giotto took a piece of charcoal and, resting his elbow on the table, with no compass to guide him, drew a perfect circle.

"Is this all I am to take?" cried the astonished messenger, when Giotto gave him the drawing of a circle.

And Giotto answered, smiling, that it was. But the Pope, looking at all of the pictures the artists had labored hard over, liked none of them. Not until he came to the perfect circle did he tell the messenger that he had, at last, found the man he wanted. The job went to Giotto. What it was, we shall never know, for the painting is gone today, but people still speak of something as being as simple as Giotto's "O."

Giotto went to Naples and painted for the king of that area. The king loved to watch the painter work and spent many hours doing just that. One hot day, as Giotto stood high on his scaffolding, without a breeze in the air, the

_____
11. Avignon (ah vee NYAWN): City in southeastern France that served as the headquarters of the pope from 1309-1377.

king, who was resting below, eating cool and juicy fruits, called lazily up to him, "Ahhhhhh . . . Giotto . . . if I were you, I would not work on such a day as this!"

Giotto laughed and answered, "No, your majesty, I would not work either, if I were *you!*"

For it was hard work to be a painter. Besides the wonderful murals, which brought painters fame and wealth, there was other work for them to do. They painted coats of arms on shields, decorated bridal chests and floats for parades and festivals. And not only did they paint and design the floats, they even painted the faces of the ladies and children who rode on them, so that they might appear as pink-cheeked and rosy-lipped as angels.

As his father on the farm, long years before, had hoped, Giotto became very rich. He married and had eight children, each one, so it was said, as homely as himself. He trained many apprentices in his workshop, and one, named Taddeo Gaddi, he adopted as his own son.

The days passed, and slowly Giotto grew to be an old man. But still he painted. He was hard at work one day when some citizens of Florence came to him and asked him to design a bell tower for the city. Although Giotto was no architect, he felt this was a great honor, and he agreed to do it. He began work at once on plans and designs for the bell tower. On it he decided to put as many of the people he had seen in his long life as he could. There would be pictures of all the different trades men followed: farming and fishing, weaving and building, masonry, carpentry and wooldying. He did not forget the sheep, the sheep he had first looked at as he learned to draw. In a shepherd's tent a man sat, guarding three nibbling sheep. A wag-tailed dog stood nearby to help. To Giotto this represented the first herdsman in all the world. One panel, too, was for the painters. There a man stood patiently and intently at work upon a panel, his well-ground colors near him in a row of little pots.

The drawings Giotto made were copied in stone by sculptors to decorate the sides of the bell tower. Huge wooden scaffoldings were built, far stronger than any that were needed for a painter, and the work on the tall stone tower was begun. For three years Giotto worked on this and nothing else. He drew and planned and directed the stonemasons and carpenters. And the tower grew and grew.

But Giotto never saw it stand tall and proud and finished. In 1337, when he was seventy-one years old, he died, and the tower was not yet done. But today, when its bell rings out across the city and up into the hills where he wandered as a shepherd boy so long ago, people say,

"The bells are ringing on Giotto's tower."

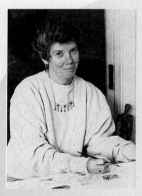

Anne Rockwell (1934–)
Childhood: Rockwell was born in Memphis, Tennessee, and grew up in many places. She once lived in New Mexico where she developed a great admiration for the Pueblo people.
Residence: She now lives in Old Greenwich, Connecticut, in a house with "a very private and secret writing room."
Profession: Rockwell is both a writer and an artist. Her own interest in art inspired her to write "The Boy Who Drew Sheep."

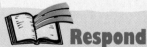

Respond

- In what ways are you like Giotto? In what ways are you different?
- Sketch a scene from your childhood.

MAKE MEANING

Explore Your Reading

Look Back (Recall)

1. What were the major events of Giotto's life?

Think It Over (Interpret)

2. Choose an event that shows Giotto's growth as an artist and explain your choice.
3. Why was Giotto such a successful and well-loved painter?
4. What do you think is Giotto's greatest achievement? Explain.

Go Beyond (Apply)

5. How did paintings reflect what medieval people valued most?

Develop Reading and Literary Skills

Analyze Historical Biography

Your chart helped you learn about the life of Giotto from this **historical biography**, the true story of a person from the past. Because the events in some historical biographies happened long ago, the writer must imagine various details. However, writers usually base what they imagine on historical evidence.

For example, the author probably did not know exactly what Cimabue and his friends were wearing when they first saw Giotto. She based her descriptions on the clothing of wealthy medieval gentlemen. In this way she made her description of the scene accurate, specific, and lively.

1. Give three other examples of details that bring the story to life and explain your choices.
2. How does actually seeing Giotto's pictures help you better understand his life?
3. A biography is a portrait in words. What picture of Giotto does the author paint? Use evidence from the selection in answering.

Ideas for Writing

Historical biographies and historical fiction, made-up stories about the past, let you imagine life in a different time. They almost make you feel as if you could "talk" with people from the past.

Apprentice's Journal Imagine that you are Giotto. Keep a daily journal that records your growth as an artist. Begin when you first come to Florence and finish with your first art commission.

Dialogue Suppose that you had an opportunity to talk with Giotto, asking him questions and telling him about today. Write the conversation that the two of you would have.

Ideas for Projects

Apprentice's Guide Research the responsibilities and the rights of apprentices during the Middle Ages. Then develop an illustrated handbook of the *dos* and *don'ts* of successful apprenticeship. [Social Studies Link]

Careers in Art Find out how people today train for a career in art. Research the different kinds of job opportunities that are available. [Art Link]

Report on Painting Ask your art teacher to help you research the artists and artwork mentioned in this story. Present your findings to your classmates, and if possible, illustrate your talk with slides or printed reproductions. [Art Link; Social Studies Link]

How Am I Doing?

Share your responses to these questions with a group of classmates:

What information about the Middle Ages did I find most interesting?

How can reading historical biographies help me in my social studies work?

Miracles by Walt Whitman
Believe in Yourself by Sandra María Esteves

What are the things that matter most to you?

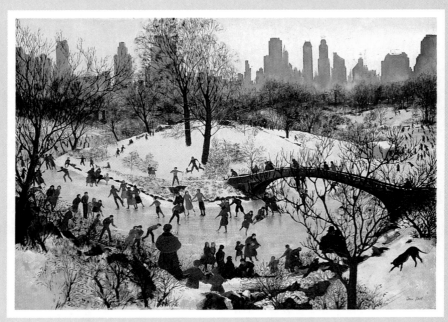

Skating in Central Park Agnes Tait, National Museum of American Art
Washington, DC/Art Resource, New York

 ## Reach Into Your Background

Imagine if everything common and ordinary suddenly vanished, except for one surviving example of each—the last six-sided snowflake, the last rose and its floating perfume, the last gritty grain of sand, the last breeze on Earth . . .

Imagining this and trying one of these activities will help you think about what matters most:

- In your journal, review your day and identify things of value—people, places, objects, ideas—both small and large. Jot down why you find these things important.
- In a group, use gestures and expressions—but not words—to suggest something you value. Have people guess what you mean.

 ## Read Actively
Identify Repetition in Poetry

Poets use **repetition**—the repeating of words, phrases, and sounds—to emphasize what matters to them. As you read poetry, identify words and sounds that haunt the poem. These repetitions are probably a clue to a central thought or feeling that also haunts the poet's mind.

In reading these two poems, look for repetitions that emphasize the meaning. Write them in your journal and say them aloud to yourself. Sometimes your ear will help you understand a phrase when your eye doesn't. See if the repetitions spark some ideas about what matters most to these poets.

Miracles

Walt Whitman

Why, who makes much of a miracle?
As to me I know of nothing else but miracles,
Whether I walk the streets of Manhattan,
Or dart my sight over the roofs of houses toward the sky,
5 Or wade with naked feet along the beach just in the edge of the water,
Or stand under trees in the woods,
Or walk by day with any one I love . . .
Or sit at table at dinner with the rest,
Or look at strangers opposite me riding in the car,
10 Or watch honeybees busy around the hive of a summer forenoon[1]
Or animals feeding in the fields,
Or birds, or the wonderfulness of insects in the air,
Or the wonderfulness of the sundown, or of stars shining so quiet and bright,
Or the exquisite[2] delicate thin curve of the new moon in spring;
15 These with the rest, one and all, are to me miracles,
The whole referring, yet each distinct and in its place.

To me every hour of the light and dark is a miracle,
Every cubic inch of space is a miracle,
Every square yard of the surface of the earth is spread with the same,
20 Every foot of the interior swarms[3] with the same.

To me the sea is a continual miracle,
The fishes that swim—the rocks—the motion of the waves—the ships with men in them.
What stranger miracles are there?

---

1. forenoon (FOR noon) *n.*: Morning.
2. exquisite (eks KWIZ it) *adj.*: Very beautiful, especially in a delicate way.
3. swarms (SWAWRMZ) *v.*: Is filled or crowded.

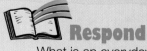 **Respond**
What is an everyday "miracle" that you know about?

Words to Know

distinct (di STINKT) *adj.*:
Different; unique (line 16)

Walt Whitman (1819–1892) is regarded today as the father of American poetry. Influenced by public speaking, opera, and news reporting, he created a new kind of poetry. Unlike formal poems with rhymes and regular beats, this free verse reflected the rhythms of American speech. It also showed the realities of American life.

Whitman himself had experienced American life in all its variety, working at different times as a printer, carpenter, teacher, and newspaper reporter.

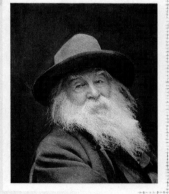

Walt Whitman
The Granger Collection, New York

Believe in Yourself

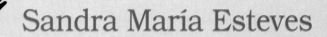

Sandra María Esteves

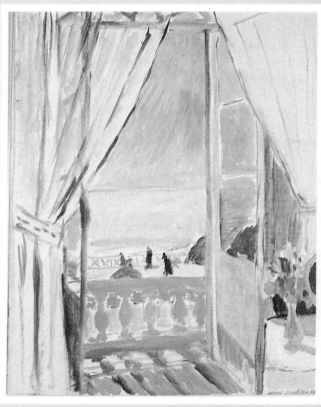

The Open Window, France Banols sur Ceze Henri Matisse
Art Resource, New York

Believe in yourself.
Be all that you can.
Look for your fate among the stars.
Imagine you are your best when being yourself
5   the best way you can.

Believe in yourself. Be all you want to be.
Open your mind, a window to the world,
different ways of thinking, seeing,
but be yourself—it's the best.

10　Become your dreams, visions to live by.
　　No matter what anyone says,
　　believe you can do it.
　　Day by day, a little at a time.
　　Be patient.

15　Believe you can find a way
　　to assemble the puzzle called life,
　　forming pictures that make some kind of sense.
　　Even when pieces fall scattered to the ground,
　　disappearing into the finite void,[1]
20　forever lost, never to be found,
　　choosing your future from those that are left,
　　like one piece from some other dimension.

　　Maybe a corner triangle shape of sky,
　　or zigzag of ocean floor with seaweed and one school of fish,
25　or maybe a centerpiece on the table in some fancy dining room,
　　or patch of window lace curtain next to flowered bouquet,
　　wind blowing through sunlight, which some artist will paint someday.
　　Or bouncing feet on the moon,
　　walking in giant moon leaps, talking moon talk,
30　deep into research in your flying laboratory.

　　Be all that you can, but believe in yourself.
　　Climb the stairway of your imagination, one step after another.
　　Growing like the leaf, blossoming into a great tree,
　　complete with squirrels, nests, universe all around.

35　Be all that you can,
　　just believe in yourself.

_____
1. **void** (VOYD) *n.*: An empty space.

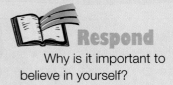

Respond

Why is it important to
believe in yourself?

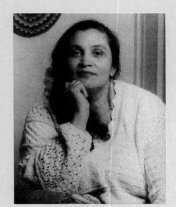

Sandra María Esteves
(1948–　) lives in New York
and is proud of her Puerto
Rican heritage. As one critic
wrote, she has "given a
voice to the Latina experience . . .
[her poetry] dares her people to celebrate their culture."

Words to Know

fate (FAYT) *n.*: Destiny; what is bound to happen
(line 3)
finite (FĪ nīt) *adj.*: Having definite, measurable
limits (line 19)

Activities
MAKE MEANING

 ## Explore Your Reading

Look Back (Recall)

1. In your own words, summarize each of these poems.

Think It Over (Interpret)

2. In his poem, why does Whitman give so many examples of miracles?
3. Does Whitman feel one miracle is greater than another? Explain.
4. What does Esteves mean when she says, "Open your mind, a window to the world, / different ways of thinking, seeing, / but be yourself — it's the best"?

Go Beyond (Apply)

5. What would these poets say to each other if they met?

 ## Develop Reading and Literary Skills

Analyze Repetition in Poetry

You've probably identified many examples of **repetition**, or the repeated use of words, phrases, and sounds, in these poems. These examples may include **alliteration**, the repetition of beginning consonant sounds in neighboring words (_W_hether I _w_alk the streets . . ."). They may also include repeated rhythms. Whenever a phrase is repeated, so is its pattern of stressed syllables ("BeLIEVE in yourSELF").

You can understand the importance of repetition in these poems if you try to imagine them without their repeated phrases. Without the words "Believe in yourself," for instance, Esteves's poem might lose its central idea and feeling of urgency.

1. Identify an example of a repetition in each of these poems and show how it contributes to the poem's meaning.
2. Rewrite a passage from one of these poems to eliminate the repetition. Then compare and contrast your passage with the original. Which is more effective? Why?

Ideas for Writing

Repeated words and phrases can also emphasize the theme of a speech or a song.

Persuasive Speech In a speech written for your classmates, tell about a person, place, or idea that matters to you. Using repeated words, phrases, and sounds, persuade your classmates to share your beliefs.

Song As you probably know, songs have repeated phrases, called refrains, that often stick in people's minds. Write a song that tells about your goals, beliefs, or values. Include a memorable refrain.

Ideas for Projects

Museum Display Many of nature's "miracles" are observable each day. Others, like rainbows and lunar eclipses, are not quite as common. Make a museum display that highlights one of nature's usual or unusual "miracles." Include illustrations, photographs, and an explanation of how the "miracle" works. [Science Link]

Class Mobile Create a class mobile—a lightweight, suspended sculpture—that expresses "visions to live by." Decide on the materials you will use, like wire, plastic, pipe cleaners, string, and papier-mâché. Then plan the mobile, construct it, and hang it in your classroom. [Art Link]

How Am I Doing?

Take a moment to discuss these questions with a partner:

How did analyzing repetition help me understand these poems better? How can I apply what I learned about repetition to other things I read?

What did these poems teach me about what matters most?

What Matters Most?

Think Critically About the Selections

All of the selections you have read in this section focus on the question "What matters most?" With a partner or a small group, complete one or two of the following activities to show what you've learned. You can write your responses in a journal or share them in discussion.

1. Choose a piece of art from this section. How do you think the artist would answer the question "What matters most?" **(Make Inferences; Provide Evidence)**

2. Choose two characters in this section who discover things that matter a great deal to them. Compare and contrast what they discover and how they discover it. **(Compare and Contrast)**

3. Imagine that two or more characters from this section meet at a party and talk about what matters most to them. Write the dialogue that would result from this meeting. **(Hypothesize)**

4. In this section, which character's or author's experiences led you to discover something about what matters most to you? Explain what you discovered and how your encounter with the character or writer led you to this discovery. **(Synthesize)**

Projects

 A Notebook of Notable People Read interviews with famous people—movie stars, sports heroes, or politicans—to get their views on what matters most. As an alternative, you can even write to

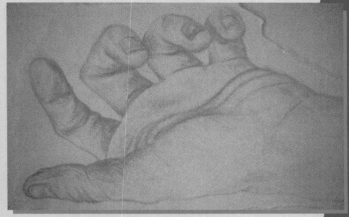

Student Art _Untitled_ Robert Wall
Overton High School, Memphis, Tennessee

them and ask them to answer this question. Collect their statements and responses in a looseleaf book, together with pictures of them.

 Collage In their work, artists use a visual "language" to say what matters most to them. Create a collage—an artwork in which pictures and bits of objects are pasted on a surface—to show what matters to you. Display your collage for your classmates. [Art Link]

 "What Matters" Survey Develop a list of things that you think might be important to people. Then interview members of your school community and ask them to rank the items on a scale of one to ten. Compile your results for presentation to your classmates. See if they agree with your findings. [Math Link]

Deciding What's Righ

In this unit, you've been reading and thinking about these important questions:

- **What Are My Choices?**
- **What Is My Responsibility to Others?**
- **What Matters Most?**

Project Menu . . . .

Other people can give you insight into what matters, but in the end you have to decide for yourself what's right. Doing projects will help you make that decision by giving you new ways of looking at choices, responsibilities, and inspirations. Here are some project ideas to choose from:

Career Day Fair You can show some of the many career choices available to students by arranging a career day. Invite people from a variety of professions and organizations to participate. Ask your guests to prepare short presentations or demonstrations of their work, and set up booths for each of them. Encourage classmates to stop at as many booths as possible. After the fair, hold a roundtable discussion on what you and your classmates learned.

Choices-and-Consequences Cartoons Create a book of humorous or serious cartoons showing different choices people make and the results of these choices. For example, you might want to humorously exaggerate the effects of littering in order to make a point. More seriously, you could show how a student's choices lead him or her to a career. Collect your cartoons in a book or display them on a bulletin board.

Way-to-Go Awards Start a program that awards students who have made your school community a better place. Accept nominations from individuals, classes, or groups. Then design award certificates and form a committee to choose the winners. You might even

From Questions to Careers

What are my choices? What is my responsibility to my friends, my family, and my community? Answers to these questions led Peter Alix to become a canine police officer. After Peter's best friend was killed in an automobile accident, his widow asked Pete to take his place in the canine training school. He honored her request and after fourteen weeks of intensive training, he and his dog Maco graduated as the number one team.

Now, Peter and Maco not only catch criminals but also do public relations work. They demonstrate the tracking and capture skills of a canine police team. Pete says, "Becoming a canine police officer is one of the best things that has happened to me. Not only can I serve my community but I have also found a wonderful partner."

What choices will you make? Make a list of what you really like to do and what you do well. Ask your school counselor and members of your community about the career choices that match your special interests and talents.

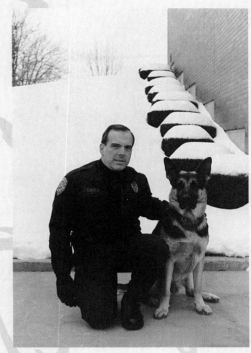

Peter Alix

check with local businesses to see if they might donate prizes. With the principal's permission, present the awards in an assembly.

Public Service Television Campaign
Develop a public service campaign to inform the community about an important issue or need. For instance, you can ask for volunteers to work at a soup kitchen or to organize a clean up of a playground. Create a series of videotaped spots that promote your issue. Then call your local television station to ask if it will air them.

Multimedia Presentation: What Matters Most?
Use different media to answer the question "What matters most?" For example, you might write a statement of belief, bring in objects that are important to you, and play audio tapes of songs that you love. However, before giving your presentation to your classmates, write a script showing how you will use the different items you have prepared.

Illustrated Book of What Matters
Working with several classmates, create a beautiful book that shows what really matters to you. Include in it pictures you draw or clip from magazines, inspiring quotations, and original or famous poems. You might even want to design it so some of the pages "pop out" at the reader. When you have finished your book, make it available to your classmates.

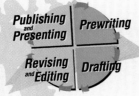

Publishing and Presenting | Prewriting
Revising and Editing | Drafting

Guided Writing

Report of Information

Reports of Information are everywhere: in encyclopedias, magazines, and newspapers, and on television and radio programs. As you write one, you'll decide what you want to research and then combine your own experiences and knowledge with information you gather from other sources: library resources, photographs, films, or interviews. Your goal is to share with others what you find out.

Guidelines • • • • • • • • • • • • • • • • •

In writing a report of information, you

- *choose a topic and develop a controlling idea.*

- *convey information accurately and effectively.*

- *engage your reader with interesting and well-organized details.*

- *elaborate with facts, examples, criteria, or personal experience.*

Prewriting

How do I choose a topic and gather information?

Choose a topic that interests you. If you care about a subject, you'll enjoy finding out more about it. Even if the report is an assignment for school, you'll probably have a choice. Don't choose what's easiest; choose what you want to know more about.

Plan your report. As you gather information, write an outline, a map, or simply a list of what you'll include. Think in terms of main idea, paragraphs, and supporting details.

Look at a variety of sources. Look at books, and magazine and newspaper articles. Skim as many as you can; choose the best ones and read them thoroughly. Take careful notes. Remember that video tapes, computers, and the Internet are sources of information.

Talk to an expert. Find someone who knows a lot about your subject and schedule an informal interview. Prepare three to five questions beforehand and bring a tape recorder.

Writing Model

Topic: Orchestras
Paragraph 1: sections
        woodwinds, brass, percussion, strings
Paragraph 2: different pitches
Paragraph 3: types of orchestras
Paragraph 4: the purpose of orchestras

This outline will help the student organize the report.

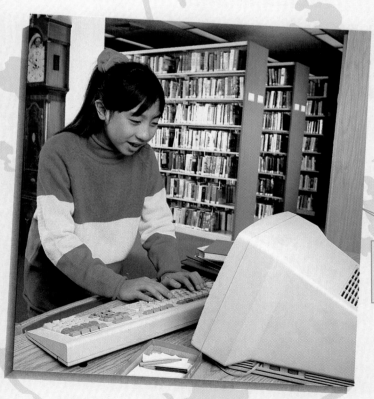

Many libraries offer on-line resources that can make research quick and fun.

Drafting

How do I get all of this information into an organized draft?

Write a one-sentence controlling idea. This doesn't have to be the first sentence of your report—in fact, it probably shouldn't be — but write one good sentence that states what your report will show.

Define unfamiliar words. If you're writing about orchestras, you may need to define *harmony, percussion, woodwind,* or *symphony.* Make definitions short but clear. Sometimes, an example will help a reader understand what you mean.

Use active voice whenever you can. Let the subject of your sentence perform the action, instead of receive it. This will bring your writing to life.

Writing Model

The instruments in the various sections are pitched in different ranges. The woodwinds, for example, have a high pitch, and the string bass has a low, rich tone. The pitches and tones of all the instruments blend together like voices singing in harmony.

> The second sentence makes the meaning of pitch clear.

> The writer uses active voice.

Revising and Editing

How can I make my report of information clearer and more interesting?

Make paragraphs intersect. One good writer's trick is to repeat a word from the last sentence of a paragraph in the first sentence of the next one. You can also use connecting words such as *in addition, similarly, next,* or *finally.*

Replace passive verbs with active verbs. Look carefully at your verbs. Make sure the subject is *doing* the action.

Writing Model

orchestra music pleases audiences.
Blending the sounds of each instrument together, the audience enjoys the orchestra music. How many instruments will you be able to identify
you hear
the next time orchestra music is heard?

> The writer has replaced a passive verb with an active one.

> The writer corrected this misplaced modifier. Originally, the sentence said the audience blended the sounds

Watch out for misplaced modifiers. If an adjective, a phrase, or a clause is separated from the word it is describing, your meaning may not be clear.

Spice up your beginning and end. Your opening sentence should grab readers' attention: a lively quotation, a question, an amazing statistic. Your ending should leave readers with a feeling of closure and satisfaction because your report has come full circle.

Checkpoints for Revision· · · · · · · · ·

- What should I add or delete to be sure the report has a clear topic and controlling idea?

- Do I move smoothly from point to point, paragraph to paragraph? How could I improve the transitions?

- What supporting details could I add to make the report more interesting to read?

Checkpoints for Editing · · · · · · · · · · ·

- Have I placed modifiers correctly in sentences?

- Have I used active voice whenever possible?

For practice in these skills, see the **Develop Your Style** lessons on the next two pages.

Publishing and Presenting

How can I share my report of information?

✔ Read your report to your classmates and answer any questions.

✔ Share your report with the person you interviewed.

✔ Print your report on one page, frame it, and display it in your school or local library.

✔ Make a class anthology entitled *What's Right for Us: Things We Care About.*

How Did I Do?

Answer these questions to see what you've learned from this assignment:

- *Did the outline help me organize my report? Would it be useful for other kinds of writing?*

- *How might learning more about certain topics help me make better decisions?*

If you like your essay, consider adding it to your portfolio.

Develop Your Style

1 Correct Misplaced or Dangling Modifiers —
How can I be sure that my phrases and clauses modify the right word?

Place a modifier as close as possible to the word it modifies. Words, phrases, and clauses that are too far from what they modify may attach themselves to the wrong word. Such **misplaced modifiers** may confuse or amuse your readers.

Avoid dangling modifers. Another incorrectly used modifer is a **dangling modifier,** which "dangles" because it modifies a word left out of the sentence.

Look at this example:

Turning the page, the overture continued.

Turning the page should modify the person playing the overture. Instead it incorrectly modifies the music itself. To correct this sentence, include information that tells who is turning the page.

Turning the page, the clarinetist continued playing the overture.

Practice correcting misplaced and dangling modifiers. Revise these sentences to get rid of misplaced or dangling modifiers.

1. The percussion instruments keep the rhythm toward the back of the stage.
2. The piccolo has a higher pitch than the tuba with its small size.
3. Confused, the kettledrum beats out the wrong rhythm.
4. Consisting of drums, cymbals, and piano, the conductor gestures wildly.

Look at your report of information. Correct any misplaced modifiers by placing the modifier as close as possible to the word it describes. Correct any dangling modifiers by inserting the word or words that go with the modifier.

Writing Model

W
With four types of stringed instruments, The string section is the heart of a symphony orchestra ~~with four types of stringed instruments~~.

> This phrase only tells how many instruments are in the string section, not in the full orchestra. To correct the sentence, the writer moved the phrase closer to the words it modifies.

Writing Model

the conductor saw that
Walking to the podium, the orchestra was ready to play.

> Notice how the confusion clears up when the writer corrects the misplaced modifier.

2 Use Active Voice

How can I make my writing crisp and direct?

Use the active voice whenever possible. Voice is the form of a verb that shows whether the subject is performing the action or having an action performed upon it. A verb is **active** if its subject performs the action. A verb is **passive** if its subject receives the action. The following examples show the same idea expressed first in the active voice and then in the passive voice.

> We bought tickets for the concert. [Subject, *We,* performs the action, *bought*]
> Tickets were bought for us. [Subject, *Tickets,* has the action performed upon it, *were bought*]

Use the active voice most of the time. Sentences with active verbs are less wordy and more direct than those with passive verbs. The sentences below tell you the same thing, but the one that uses the active voice is briefer and crisper.

> **Active:** Jim opened the program.
>
> **Passive:** The program was opened by Jim.

Writing Model

The conductor sets

∧The mood and interpretation of a piece of music ~~is set by the conductor. The conductor's lead~~

Each musician follows the conductor's lead.

∧~~is followed by each musician in the orchestra~~. Without the conductor, an orchestra could easily fall apart.

Some situations call for use of the passive voice. Use the passive voice when you want to emphasize the receiver of the action rather than the doer of the action or when you do not know who performs the action. For example, this sentence emphasizes the solo and not the student:

> The flute solo was played by a high school student.

Practice using the active voice. Revise these sentences so they are in the active voice.

1. The main theme of the concerto was played first by the woodwinds.
2. The lively melody was picked up by the violins and violas.
3. They were followed by the entire orchestra.

Look at your report of information. Have you used active voice wherever you could? Change your passive verbs to active ones to keep your writing forceful and direct.

Book News

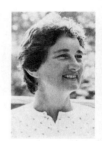

• • • • • • • • • • • Deciding

Featured Review

The Master Puppeteer
by Katherine Paterson

Books can take you to different times and far-away places. *The Master Puppeteer* takes you all the way back to medieval Japan. Osaka, where the story is set, was a difficult city in which to be poor. Food was scarce and taxes were high, making life in a poor famiy tough. However, roaming the streets of Osaka, a mysterious bandit called Saburo robbed the rich to help the poor.

Jiro, the son of a poor puppet maker, is

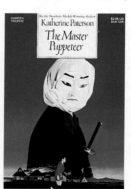

apprenticed to the master of the local puppet show, Yoshida. As the story unfolds, Jiro struggles to keep his parents and friend out of danger. Jiro also works to uncover the true identity of Saburo. When he discovers the truth, he has to make an important decision. Should he tell, or keep the robber's identity secret?

The Master Puppeteer is a story of adventure, mystery, and the struggle for survival in a time of social injustice.

Introducing the Author

Katherine Paterson (1932–) was born in China and educated in that country, the United States, and Japan. She says that she became a writer without really planning to be one. "I turned to writing fiction because that is what I most enjoy reading."

Paterson often gets ideas for her writing from her own children. She says, "When my (adopted) daughter Lin was concerned about who her biological parents might be, and there was no way I could help her find out about them, I wrote a book instead." That book was Paterson's first novel, *The Sign of the Chrysanthemum*.

The author dedicated *The Master Puppeteer* to her daughter Mary, and the two boys in the book both resemble her older son, John. All four of her children read her manuscripts and make suggestions, which she doesn't always take!

Pass It On: Student Choices

The True Confessions of Charlotte Doyle by Avi

Reviewed by Christina Casanova, McKinley Classic Jr. Academy, St. Louis, Missouri

To join her family, Charlotte crosses the Atlantic by ship in 1832. The captain is mean and the crew wants to mutiny. I like the attitude of Charlotte Doyle, the main character of this book. She is independent, a quality she needs to survive her experiences. Her will to live helps her, too. The story is very eventful and exciting. It also ends well; and what good is a book that ends wrong?

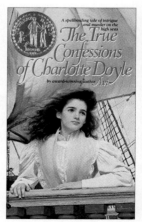

Journal

What's Right • • • • • • • •

The Red Pony
by John Steinbeck

**Reviewed by Andrew Lippman,
Thomas A. Blake Middle School,
Medfield, Massachusetts**

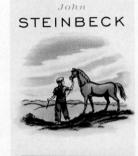

This book is the story of Jody, a boy learning about life and death on a ranch in California. What I liked most was the way the author expressed the feelings of the characters. I could *feel* the emotions of every character.

I, Juan de Pareja
by Elizabeth Borton de Treviño

**Reviewed by Megan Wiseman, Eisenhower Middle School,
New Berlin, Wisconsin**

I like to draw and have always wanted to be an artist. Juan painted in secret but couldn't show his

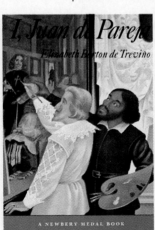

paintings since he was a slave. He decided to tell his master Diego his secret. There was a line in the afterword that said, " . . . those two, who began in youth as master and slave, continued as companions in their maturity and ended as equals and as friends." It brings it all together in one powerful sentence.

Read On: More Choices

Chico Mendes: Defender of the Rain Forest **by Joanna J. Burch**

What Happened at Hamelin **by Gloria Skurzynski**

Jazz: My Music, My People **by Morgan Monceaux**

The Well **by Mildred Taylor**

Share the Fun

A Book Bunch Find a book you and several classmates want to read. Decide how many times the members of your book bunch want to meet about the book and assign chapters to read before each session.

Readers Theater With members of your group, prepare and perform a readers theater presentation. Readers theater is not acting; it's a dramatic reading. Some members become the characters and read their words and thoughts to the audience. A narrator reads other material. You don't have to memorize the words. You suggest the character or the meaning of the passage vocally by reading with feeling.

A Book Postcard Send a postcard from the main character of your book to readers. Draw a picture or paste a magazine illustration on the back side of the postcard to suggest an important place depicted in the book. As the main character, write a message to readers that shares your reaction to an important event in the book. Postmark the card by using the time and place that would be right for the book. Create an appropriate stamp, too.

GLOSSARY

Pronunciation Key

The vocabulary and footnotes in this textbook are respelled to aid pronunciation. A syllable in CAPITAL LETTERS receives the most stress. The key below lists the letters used for respelling. It includes examples of words using each sound and shows how the words would be respelled.

Symbol	Example	Respelled	Symbol	Example	Respelled
a	hat, cat	hat, cat	oh	no, toe	noh, toh
ay	pay, ape	pay, ayp	oo	look, pull, put	look, pool, poot
ah	hot, stop	haht, stahp	oy	boil, toy	boyl, toy
aw	law, all, horn	law, awl, hawrn	oo	ooze, tool, crew	ooz, tool, croo
			ow	plow, out	plow, owt
e	met, elf, ten	met, elf, ten			
ee	bee, eat, flea	bee, eet, flee	u	up, cut, flood	up, cut, flud
er	learn, sir, fur	lern, ser, fer	yoo	few, use	fyoo, yooz
i	is	fit	uh	a in ago	uh GO
ī	mile, sigh	mīle sīgh		e in agent	AY juhnt
				i in sanity	SAN uh tee
				o in compress	kuhm PRES
				u in focus	FOH kuhs

A

adjoining (uh JOY ning) *adj.*: Next to; near
ajar (uh JAR) *adj.*: Open
alchemist (AL kuh mist) *n.*: Someone who practiced alchemy, a medieval form of chemistry. Alchemists tried to turn common metals into gold
annual (AN yoo uhl) *adj.*: Happening every year
anxious (ANK shuhs) *adj.*: Worried, uneasy in mind
apothecary (uh PAHTH uh ker ee) *n.*: Pharmacist; druggist
apparent (uh PAR uhnt) *adj.*: Seeming to be, but is perhaps not
apparition (ap uh RISH uhn) *n.*: Ghost
apprentice (uh PREN tis) *n.*: One who receives financial support and instruction in a trade in return for work
aspiration (as puhr AY shun) *n.*: Strong wish, hope, or ambition
astonish (uh STAHN ish) *v.*: Amaze
audible (AW duh buhl) *adj.*: Loud enough to be heard

B

banister (BAN is tuhr) *n.*: Railing along a staircase
battered (BAT uhrd) *adj.*: Damaged; worn out
beacon (BEE kuhn) *n.*: Shining example
betrothal (bee TROH thuhl) *n.*: Engagement to be married
blackmail (BLAK mayl) *v.*: Threaten to tell something harmful about someone unless certain conditions are met
bodega (boh DAY guh) *n.*: A small grocery store serving a Latino neighborhood
burnish (BER nish) *v.*: To polish

C

calico (KAL uh koh) *n.*: A coarse and cheap cloth
candy (KAN dee) *v.*: Coat with sugar
catalyst (CAT uh list) *n.*: An inspiration; a substance that causes a chemical change when added to something but is not changed itself
classified document (KLAS i fid DAHK yoo ment) *n.*: Secret government paper
cohort (KOH hawrt) *n.*: Fellow worker, associate
comforter (KUHM fuhr tuhr) *n.*: A long, woolen scarf
commission (kuh MISH en) *v.*: Hire
compulsion (kuhm PUHL shun) *n.*: A driving, irresistible force
concentration camp (kahn sen TRA shun KAMP) *n.*: A prison camp where Nazis held Jews and others during World War II
concessionaire (kuhn sesh uh NAYR) *n.*: Business person
confront (kuhn FRUHNT) *v.*: Stand up against
contamination (kuhn tam i NAY shun) *n.*: Pollution by poison or other dangerous substances
corrode (kuh ROHD) *v.*: Rust; wear away
curdle (KUR duhl) *adj.*: Thicken, clot

D

deliquesce (DEL uh kwes) *v.*: Melt away
destitute (DES tuh toot) *adj.*: Living in complete poverty
disdainful (dis DAYN fuhl) *adj.*: Showing arrogance or scorn for someone considered beneath oneself
dispel (di SPEL) *v.*: Scatter and drive away, make vanish

disperse (di SPERS) *v.*: Break up, scatter in all directions

distinct (di STINKT) *adj.*: Different; unique

E

ermine (UR muhn) *adj.*: From the northern European weasel

exhilarating (eg zil uh RAYT ing) *v.*: Exciting; lively

exquisite (eks KWIZ it) *adj.*: Very beautiful, especially in a delicate way

F

farthing (FAHR thing) *n.*: A small British coin

fate (FAYT) *n.*: Destiny; what is bound to happen

fifer (FĪ fuhr) *n.*: Musician playing small flute

finite (FĪ nīt) *adj.*: Having definite, measurable limits

fledgling (FLEJ ling) *n.*: Young birds that have just grown the feathers needed for flying

forenoon (FOR noon) *n.*: Morning

forfeit (FOR fit) *v.*: Give up or lose something

G

gawking (GAWK ing) *adj.*: Staring

glut (GLUHT) *v.*: Given more than is needed or wanted

gnarled (NAHRLD) *adj.*: Knotty and twisted

gnaw (NAW) *v.*: Bite or wear away bit by bit

grieve (GREEV) *v.*: Feel deep sadness or grief

gurney (GER nee) *n.*: A stretcher on wheels

I

idle reverie (ĪD uhl REV er ee) *n.*: Day dreaming

implore (im PLAWR) *v.*: Ask or beg earnestly

impromptu (im PRAHMP too) *adj.*: Unscheduled, unplanned

impudently (im PYOO duhnt lee) *adv.*: Shamelessly, disrespectfully

incense (IN sens) *n.*: Any of various substances that produce a pleasant odor when burned

indignant (in DIG nuhnt) *adj.*: Angry about something that seems unfair or mean

inequity (in EK wuh tee) *n.*: Unfairness; instance that reveals injustice

inheritance (in HER i tuhns) *n.*: A gift passed from one generation to the next

instinct (in STINKT) *n.*: A way of acting that is natural to people and animals from birth, not learned

intently (in TENT lee) *adv.*: Purposefully, carefully

intercom (IN tuhr kahm) *n.*: A communication system used in apartment buildings

internship (IN tuhrn ship) *n.*: A job that helps young people learn about careers by training in specific businesses

K

koppie (KAHP ee) *n.*: In South Africa, a small hill

L

lattice (LAT uhs) *n.*: A structure of crossed strips of wood or metal, used as a support

live wire (LĪV WĪR) *n.*: A wire with electricity running through it, which is potentially dangerous to touch

lute (LOOT) *n.*: An old-fashioned stringed instrument like a guitar

lyre (LĪR) *n.*: Harp

M

mangy (MAYN gee) *adj.*: Dirty

maul (MAWL) *v.*: Attack, handle roughly

meager (MEE guhr) *adj.*: Of poor quality, small in amount

memento (muh MEN toh) *n.*: Souvenir; keepsake; object to remind a person of something

menace (MEN uhs) *v.*: Threaten

mica (MĪ kuh), **feldspar** (FELD spahr), **hornblende** (HAWRN blend) *n.*: Common minerals found in rocks

mine skip (MĪN SKIP) *n.*: Small, open cart in which miners and materials travel up and down mine shafts

minimum wage (MIN i mum WAJ) *n.*: The lowest rate of pay allowed by law

misanthrope (MIS uhn throhp) *n.*: A person who hates or distrusts everyone

morose (muh ROHS) *adj.*: Gloomy, ill-tempered

mural (MYOO ruhl) *n.*: Image painted on a wall

musty (MUS tee) *adj.*: Having a stale, moldy smell

N

neglect (ni GLEKT) *n.*: Little attention

O

ominous (AHM uh nuhs) *adj.*: Threatening, frightening

P

parchment (PARCH muhnt) *n.*: The skin of a sheep or goat that has been prepared so that it can be written or painted on

penance (PEN uhns) *n.*: Any suffering a person takes on to show sorrow for wrongdoing

perch (PERCH) *n.*: A resting place, especially a high or insecure one

philosophy (fuh LAHS uh fee) *n.*: A set of beliefs

plantain (PLAN tuhn) *n.*: A kind of banana plant bearing a fruit that is cooked and eaten as a vegetable

plausible (PLAW zuh buhl) *adj.*: Seemingly true, acceptable or honest, but open to some doubt

ponder (PAHN duhr) *v.*: Think deeply about; consider carefully

ponderous (PAHN duhr uhs) *adj.*: Very heavy, bulky

pound (POWND) *n.*: British currency

prawn (PRAWN) *n.*: A shellfish that is like a large shrimp

preserve (pree ZURV) *v.*: Save in a good condition; keep

prey (PRAY) *v.*: Hunt other animals for food

proposal (pruh POH zuhl) *n.*: An offer or suggestion

pylon (PĪ lahn) *n.*: Towerlike structure

Q

quivering (KWIV uh ring) *v.*: Shaking, trembling

R

rancid (RAN sid) *adj.*: Spoiled and bad-smelling

rapt (RAPT) *adj.*: Giving complete attention, totally carried away by something

rational (RASH uh nuhl) *adj.*: Logical, able to reason

realign (ree uh LĪN) *v.*: Readjust the parts so they work well together

relate (ri LAYT) *v.*: Tell

remorse (rih MAWRS) *n.*: Sorrow, regret for previous action

reputation (re pyoo TAY shun) *n.*: What people generally think about the character of someone else

requite (ree KWĪT) *v.*: Return; reward

resent (ree ZENT) *v.*: Feel bitter, hurt, or angry about something

reveler (REV uh ler) *n.*: Person who is celebrating

revelry (REV uhl ree) *n.*: Celebration, noisy merry-making

rind (RĪND) *n.*: Tough outer layer or skin

S

sacrifice (SAK ruh fīs) *n.*: Loss, giving up one thing for the sake of something else

scaffolding (SKAF uhl ding) *n.*: A framework put up to support workers while they are building, reparing or painting something

scalawag (SKAL uh wag) *n.*: Person who causes trouble, scoundrel

scour (SKOWR) *v.*: Clean by rubbing vigorously

scrim (SKRIM) *n.*: A light, semi-transparent curtain

seize (SEEZ) *v.*: Take hold of suddenly; grasp

severe (suh VEER) *adj.*: Harsh

shrine (SHRĪN) *n.*: A place of worship

skein (SKAYN) *n.*: Loose thick coil

solemnize (SAHL uhm nīz) *v.*: Honor or remember

spasm (SPAZ uhm) *n.*: A short, sudden burst

specter (SPEK tur) *n.*: Ghost

squander (SKWAHN duhr) *v.*: Waste; spend foolishly

subtle (SUH tuhl) *adj.*: Sly; not open or direct

summit (SUHM it) *n.*: The highest point, the top

supervise (SOO puhr vīz) *v.*: Direct or manage, oversee

surpass (ser PAS) *v.*: To be better than; to go beyond a limit

swarm (SWAWRM) *v.*: To fill or crowd

T

tawdry (TAW dree) *adj.*: Cheap and showy, gaudy

tenement (TEN uh mint) *n.*: An old, run down apartment house

tentatively (TEN tuh tiv lee) *adv.*: Hesitantly, with uncertainty

threadbare (THRED bayr) *adj.*: Worn, shabby

V

vault (VAWLT) *n.*: A safe for keeping valuables; *v.*: jump over

veld (VELT) *n.*: Open grassy country with few bushes and almost no trees

veteran (VET uhr uhn) *adj.*: Experienced

void (VOYD) *n.*: Total emptiness

vow (VOW) *v.*: Promise, pledge

W

wattle (WAHT uhl) *n.*: Framework or pile of sticks, branches, etc

wither (WITH uhr) *adj.*: Dry up

Y

yield (YEELD) *v.*: Give way to pressure or force

Index of Fine Art

Index of Authors and Titles

Page numbers in italics refer to biographical information.

Index of Skills

Literary Terms

Biography, H68, H74, H155
  Analyze Historical, H155
  Evaluate, H74
  Make Inferences About the Subject of, H68
Character Development, H100, H122
  Observe in Drama, H100
  Understand Character Development and Theme, H122
Characters, H20, H29
  Draw Conclusions About, H20
  Understand Theme Through, H29
Conflict, H38, H41, H78
  Analyze in a Folk Tale, H41
  Gather Evidence About, H38
  Identify in Drama, H78
Drama, H36, H76, H78, H99, H100
  Analyze Plot in, H99
  Dialogue, H76
  Identify Conflicts in, H78
  Looking at, H76
  Observe Character Development in, H100
  Plot, H76
  Script, H76
  Stage Directions, H76
Essay, H30, H34, H134, H139
  Analyze a Reflective Essay, H139
  Connect an Essay to Your Experience, H30
  Identify Elements of a Reflective Essay, H134
  Respond to a Personal Essay, H34
Exaggeration, H16
Folk Tales, H36, H41, H42, H46
  Analyze Conflict in, H41
  Identify Cause and Effect in, H42
  Looking at, H36
  Trickster, H36
  Understand Metamorphosis in, H46
Humor, H6, H19
  Appreciate in Poetry, H19
Images, H57
  Examine in Poetry, H57
Plot, H76, H99
  Analyze in Drama, H99
Poetic Forms, H143
Poetry, H19, H54, H57, H140, H156, H160
  Analyze Repetition in, H160
  Appreciate Humor in, H19
  Examine Images in , H57
  Identify Repetition in, H156
  Recognize Forms in, H140
  Visualize Images in, H54
Setting, H124, H133
  Appreciate, H133
  Identify Details of, H124
Story, H48
  Make Predictions About, H48
Surprise Ending, H53
Suspense, H8, H15
  Analyze, H15
  Identify Details that Create, H8
Symbols, H58, H67
  Analyze, H67
  Gather Evidence About, H58
Theme, H29, H122
  Understand Character Development and, H122

Understand Through Character, H29

Reading and Thinking Skills

Analyze, H75
Apply, H75
Compare and Contrast, H75, H161
Connect, H3, H30, H144
  Essay to Your Experience, H30
  Literature to Social Studies, H144
Draw Conclusions, H20, H35
  About Characters, H20
Evaluate, H35, H74
  Biography, H74
Gather Evidence, H38, H58
  About a Conflict, H38
  About Symbols, H58
Hypothesize, H35, H75, H161
Make Inferences, H35, H68, H161
  About the Subject of a Biography, H68
Predict, H3, H48
  About a Story, H48
Preview, H2
Provide Evidence, H35, H161
Recognize Forms in Poetry, H140
Respond, H3, H34
  to a Personal Essay, H34
Summarize, H35
Synthesize, H35, H75, H161
Visualize Images, H3, H54
  In Poetry, H54

Ideas for Writing

Anecdote, H29
Apprentice's Journal, H155
Baby-sitter's Journal, H15
Biographical Sketch, H74
Casting Memo, H122
Character's Farewell, H46
Company Report, H67
Comparison and Contrast, H6
Credo Monologue, H133
Dialogue, H155
Double Eulogy, H122
Dramatic Scene, H99
Editorial, H15
Eulogy, H29
Fairy Tale, H6
Fantasy, H46
Feature Story, H19
Folk Tale, H41, H74
Graduation Speech, H139
How-to Manual, H139
Interpretation, H143
Legal Brief, H41
Letter to the Editor, H57
Limerick, H143
Monologue, H67
Personal Essay, H34
Personal Letter, H99
Persuasive Speech, H160
Poem, H19, H57 Report of Information (Guided Writing Lesson),   H164
Science-Fiction Story, H53
Short Story, H34
Song, H160
Stage Set Design, H133
TV Feature Story, H53

Ideas for Projects

Animal Rescue and Protection, H67
Annotated Movie Guide, H57
Apprentice's Guide, H155
Audio Presentation of the Blues, H133
Career Day Fair, H162
Career Panel, H143
Careers in Art, H155
Character Profile, H122
Checklist, H15
Choices-and-Consequences Cartoons, H162
Class Mobile, H160
Collage, H19, H161
Community Participation, H74
Consumer Report, H143
Dance, H41, H139
Environmental Issues Project, H75
Folk-Tale Anthology, H41
Goals Book, H34
History of Christmas, H122
Holiday Research, H122
Holocaust Report, H29
How-to Fair, H74
I-Search Project, H35
Illustrated Book of What Matters, H163
Illustrated Report, H15
Invitation to a Holiday Celebration, H99
Landscape, H46
Leadership Training, H139
Mobile, H75
Multimedia Presentation: Choices, H35
Museum Display, H160
Notebook of Notable People, H161
Oral Report on Homelessness, H133
Personal Interview With Career Professionals, H35
Poster Campaign, H53
Precious Gems Presentation, H6
Proposal Chart, H74
Public Service Television Campaign, H163
Readers Theater, H6
Report on Painting, H155
Responsibility Survey, H75
Science Report, H29
Set Design, H99
Song, H34
South African Background, H67
Space Capsule, H133
Speaker from the Community, H53
Statistical Report of the Environment, H19
Teens Who Made a Difference, H67
Video/Computer Game, H53
Way-to-Go Awards, H162
Weather Report, H46
What Matters in Multimedia, H162
"What Matters" Survey, H161
Zoo Report, H57

Student Review Board

Acharya, Arundhathi
Cecelia Snyder Middle School
Bensalem, Pennsylvania

Adkisson, Grant
McClintock Middle School
Charlotte, North Carolina

Akuna, Kimberly
Harriet Eddy Middle School
Elk Grove, California

Amdur, Samantha
Morgan Selvidge Middle School
Ballwin, Missouri

Arcilla, Richard
Village School
Closter, New Jersey

Arredondo, Marcus
Keystone School
San Antonio, Texas

Auten, Kristen
Bernardo Heights Middle School
San Diego, California

Backs, Jamie
Cross Keys Middle School
Florissant, Missouri

Baldwin, Katie
Bonham Middle School
Temple, Texas

Barber, Joanna
Chenery School
Belmont, Massachusetts

Bates, Maureen
Chestnut Ridge Middle School
Sewell, New Jersey

Bates, Meghan
Chestnut Ridge Middle School
Sewell, New Jersey

Beber, Nick
Summit Middle School
Dillon, Colorado

Becker, Jason
Hicksville Middle School
Hicksville, New York

Belfon, Loreal
Highland Oaks Middle School
Miami, Florida

Belknap, Jessica
Hughes Middle School
Long Beach, California

Bennet, Joseph
Conner Middle School
Hebron, Kentucky

Birke, Lori
LaSalle Springs Middle School
Glencoe, Missouri

Bleichrodt, Angela
Beulah School
Beulah, Colorado

Block, Kyle
Hall-McCarter Middle School
Blue Springs, Missouri

Brendecke, Sarah Grant
Baseline Middle School
Boulder, Colorado

Brooks, Beau
Cresthill Middle School
Highlands Ranch, Colorado

Bruder, Jennifer
Nipher Middle School
Kirkwood, Missouri

Brunsfeld, Courtney
Moscow Junior High School
Moscow, Idaho

Burnett, Joseph
Markham Intermediate School
Placerville, California

Burrows, Tammy
Meadowbrook Middle School
Orlando, Florida

Calles, Miguel
Lennox Middle School
Lennox, California

Casanova, Christina
McKinley Classic Junior Academy
St. Louis, Missouri

Ceaser, Cerena
Templeton Middle School
Templeton, California

Chapman, Jon
Black Butte Middle School
Shingletown, California

Cho, Hwa
Miami Lakes Middle School
Miami Lakes, Florida

Chu, Rita
Orange Grove Middle School
Hacienda Heights, California

Church, John
Nathan Hale Middle School
Norwalk, Conneticut

Clouse, Melissa Ann
Happy Valley Elementary School
Anderson, California

Colbert, Ryanne
William H. Crocker School
Hillsborough, California

Crucet, Jennine
Miami Lakes Middle School
Miami Lakes, Florida

Culp, Heidi
Eastern Christian Middle School
Wyckoff, New Jersey

Cummings, Amber
Pacheco Elementary School
Redding, California

Curran, Christopher
Cresthill Middle School
Highlands Ranch, Colorado

D'Angelo, Samantha
Cresthill Middle School
Highlands Ranch, Colorado

D'Auria, Jeffrey
Nyack Middle School
Nyack, New York

D'Auria, Katherine
Upper Nyack Elementary School
Upper Nyack, New York

D'Auria, Patrick
Nyack Middle School
Nyack, New York

Daughtride, Katharyne
Lakeview Middle School
Winter Garden, Florida

Donato, Bridget
Felix Festa Junior High School
New City, New York

Donato, Christopher
Felix Festa Junior High School
New City, New York

Dress, Brian
Hall-McCarter Middle School
Blue Springs, Missouri

Drilling, Sarah
Milford Junior High School
Milford, Ohio

Fernandez, Adrian
Shenandoah Middle School
Coral Gables, Florida

Flores, Amanda
Orange Grove Middle School
Hacienda Heights, California

Flynn, Patricia
Camp Creek Middle School
College Park, Georgia

Ford, Adam
Cresthill Middle School
Highlands Ranch, Colorado

Fowler, Sabrina
Camp Creek Middle School
College Park, Georgia

Fox, Anna
Georgetown School
Georgetown, California

Freeman, Ledon
Atlanta, Georgia

Frid-Nielsen, Snorre
Branciforte Elementary School
Santa Cruz, California

Frosh, Nicole
Columbia Middle School
Aurora, Colorado

Gerretson, Bryan
Marshfield Junior High School
Marshfield, Wisconsin

Gillis, Shalon Michelle
Wagner Middle School
Philadelphia, Pennsylvania

Gonzales, Michael
Kitty Hawk Junior High School
Universal City, Texas

Goodman, Andrew
Richmond School
Hanover, New Hampshire

Granberry, Kemoria
Riviera Middle School
Miami, Florida

Groppe, Karissa
McCormic Junior High School
Cheyenne, Wyoming

Hadley, Michelle
Hopkinton Middle School
Hopkinton, Massachusetts

Hall, Katie
C.R. Anderson Middle School
Helena, Montana

Hamilton, Tim
Columbia School
Redding, California

Hawkins, Arie
East Norriton Middle School
Norristown, Pennsylvania

Hawkins, Jerry
Carrollton Junior High School
Carrollton, Missouri

Hayes, Bridget
Point Fermin Elementary School
San Pedro, California

Heinen, Jonathan
Broomfield Heights Middle School
Broomfield, Colorado

Hibbard, Erin
Willard Grade Center
Ada, Oklahoma

Hinners, Katie
Spaulding Middle School
Loveland, Ohio

Houston, Robert
Allamuchy Township Elementary
Allamuchy, New Jersey

Huang, Kane
Selridge Middle School
Ballwin, Missouri

Hudson, Vanessa
Bates Academy
Detroit, Michigan

Hutchison, Erika
C.R. Anderson Middle School
Helena, Montana

Hykes, Melissa
Meadowbrook Middle School
Orlando, Florida

Jackson, Sarah Jane
Needles Middle School
Needles, California

Jigarjian, Kathryn
Weston Middle School
Weston, Massachusetts

Johnson, Becky
Wheatland Junior High School
Wheatland, Wyoming

Johnson, Bonnie
West Middle School
Colorado Springs, Colorado

Johnson, Courtney
Oak Run Elementary School
Oak Run, California

Jones, Mary Clara
Beulah Middle School
Beulah, Colorado

Jones, Neil
Central School
Chillicothe, Missouri

Juarez, Sandra
Adams City Middle School
Thornton, Colorado

Juarez, Karen
Rincon Middle School
Escondito, California

Karas, Eleni
Our Lady of Grace
Encino, California

King, Autumn
Roberts Paideia Academy
Cincinnati, Ohio

Kossenko, Anna
Plantation Middle School
Plantation, Florida

Kurtz, Rachel
Paul Revere Middle School
Los Angeles, California

Lambino, Victoria
Henry H. Wells Middle School
Brewster, New York

Lamour, Katleen
Highland Oaks Middle School
North Miami Beach, Florida

Larson, Veronica
McClintock Middle School
Charlotte, North Carolina

Liao, Wei-Cheng
Nobel Middle School
Northridge, California

Lightfoot, Michael
Mission Hill Middle School
Santa Cruz, California

Lippman, Andrew
Thomas A. Blake Middle School
Medfield, Massachusetts

Lo, Melissa
Lincoln Middle School
Santa Monica, California

Lopez, Eric
Irvine Intermediate School
Costa Mesa, California

Lowery, Ry-Yon
East Norriton Middle School
Norristown, Pennsylvania

Macias, Edgar
Teresa Hughes Elementary School
Cudahy, California

Madero, Vanessa
Mathew J. Brletic Elementary
Parlier, California

Mandel, Lily
Mission Hill Junior High School
Santa Cruz, California

Manzano, Elizabeth Josephine
Hillside Elementary School
San Bernardino, California

Marentes, Crystal-Rose
Orange Grove Middle School
Hacienda Heights, California

Martinez, Desiree
Wheatland Junior High School
Wheatland, Wyoming

Massey, Drew
Union 6th and 7th Grade Center
Tulsa, Oklahoma

Matson, Josh
Canyon View Junior High School
Orem, Utah

Maxcy, Donald, Jr.
Camp Creek Middle School
Atlanta, Georgia

Maybruch, Robyn
Middle School 141
Riverdale, New York

Mayer, Judith
Burlingame Intermediate School
Burlingame, California

McCarter, Jennifer
Washburn School
Cincinnati, Ohio

McCarthy, Megan
Richmond School
Hanover, New Hampshire

McCombs, Juanetta
Washburn School
Cincinnati, Ohio

McGann, Kristen
Orange Grove Middle School
Hacienda Heights, California

McKelvey, Steven
Providence Christian Academy
Atlanta, Georgia

McQuary, Megan
CCA Baldi Middle School
Philadelphia, Pennsylvania

Mercier, Jared
Marshfield Junior High School
Marshfield, Wisconsin

Merrill, Nick
Windham Middle School
Windham, Maine

Miller, Catherine
Neil Armstrong Junior High School
Levittown, Pennsylvania

Miller, Kristen
Marina Village Junior High
El Dorado Hills, California

Montgomery, Tyler
North Cow Creek School
Palo Cedro, California

Mueller, Jessica
Spaulding Middle School
Loveland, Ohio

Mueler, John
St. Catherine School
Milwaukee, Wisconsin

Mulligan, Rebecca
Herbert Hoover Middle School
Oklahoma City, Oklahoma

Murgel, John
Beulah School
Beulah, Colorado

Murphy, Mathew
St. Wenceslaus School
Omaha, Nebraska

Neeley, Alex
Allamuchy Township School
Allamuchy, New Jersey

Nelsen-Smith, Nicole Marie
Branciforte Elementary
Santa Cruz, California

Ogle, Sarah
Redlands Middle School
Grand Junction, Colorado

Ozeryansky, Svetlana
C.C.A. Baldi Middle School
Philadelphia, Pennsylvania

Pacheco, Vicky
East Whittier Middle School
Whittier, California

Paddack, Geoffrey
Ada Junior High School
Ada, Oklahoma

Palombi, Stephanie
Marina Village Middle School
Cameron Park, California

Panion, Stephanie
Pitts Middle School
Pueblo, Colorado

Parks, Danny
West Cottonwood Junior High School
Cottonwood, California

Parriot, Cassandra
Orange Grove Middle School
Hacienda Heights, California

Paulson, Christina
Jefferson Middle School
Rocky Ford, Colorado

Perez, Iscura
Charles Drew Middle School
Los Angeles, California

Pratt, Lisa
Nottingham Middle Community Education Center
St. Louis, Missouri

Raggio, Jeremiah
Eagleview Middle School
Colorado Springs, Colorado

Raines, Angela
McKinley Classical Academy
St. Louis, Missouri

Ramadan, Mohammad
Ada Junior High School
Ada, Oklahoma

Ramiro, Leah
Magruder Middle School
Torrance, California

Raymond, Elizabeth
Julia A. Traphagen School
Waldwick, New Jersey

Recinos, Julie
Riviera Middle School
Miami, Florida

Reese, Andrea
Moscow Junior High
Moscow, Idaho

Reiners, Andrew
Redlands Middle School
Grand Junction, Colorado

Riddle, Katy
Willard Elementary School
Ada, Oklahoma

Rippe, Chris
La Mesa Junior High School
Santa Clarita, California

Robinson, Barbara
Wagner Middle School
Philadelphia, Pennsylvania

Rochford, Tracy
Louis Armstrong Middle School/IS 227
East Elmhurst, New York

Rodriguez, Ashley
John C. Martinez Junior High School
Parlier, California

Rowe, Michael
Washington Middle School
Long Beach, California

Sayles, Nichole
Hall McCarter Middle School
Blue Springs, Missouri

Schall, Harvest
Castle Rock Elementary School
Castella, California

Schellenberg, Katie
Corpus Christi School
Pacific Palisades, California

Schmees, Katherine
Milford Junior High School
Milford, Ohio

Schned, Paul
Richmond School
Hanover, New Hampshire

Schneider, Jennie
Parkway West Middle School
Chesterfield, Missouri

Scialanga, Michelle
Taylor Middle School
Millbrae, California

Shye, Kathryn
Happy Valley Elementary School
Anderson, California

Sirikulvadhana, Tiffany
Orange Grove Middle School
Hacienda Heights, California

Smetak, Laura
Orange Grove Middle School
Hacienda Heights, California

Smith, Shannon
Mary Putnam Henck Intermediate School
Lake Arrowhead, California

Smith-Paden, Patricia
Chappelow Middle School
Evans, Colorado

Sones, Mandy
Knox Junior High School
The Woodlands, Texas

Song, Sarah
Orange Grove Middle School
Hacienda Heights, California

Souza, Molly
Georgetown School
Georgetown, California

Stewart, Larry
Windsor Elementary School
Cincinnati, Ohio

Stites, Aaron
Redlands Middle School
Grand Junction, Colorado

Sturzione, James Van Duyn
Glen Rock Middle School
Glen Rock, New Jersey

Sundberg, Sarah
Milford Junior High School
Milford, Ohio

Swan, Tessa
Pacheco Elementary School
Redding, California

Swanson, Kurt
Allamuchy Elementary School
Allamuchy, New Jersey

Swihart, Bruce
Redlands Middle School
Grand Junction, Colorado

Syron, Christine
Nottingham Middle Community Education Center
St. Louis, Missouri

Taylor, Cody
Bella Vista Elementary School
Bella Vista, California

Thomas, Jennifer
Hoover Middle School
San Jose, California

Thompson, Robbie
Hefner Middle School
Oklahoma City, Oklahoma

Todd, Wanda
Hampton Middle School
Detroit, Michigan

Torning, Fraser
Allamuchy Elementary School
Allamuchy, New Jersey

Torres, Erica
Truman Middle School
Albuquerque, New Mexico

Tyroch, Melissa
Bonham Middle School
Temple, Texas

Ulibarri, Shavonne
John C. Martinez Junior High School
Parlier, California

Vanderham, Lynsey
Eagleview Middle School
Colorado Springs, Colorado

Vemula, Suni
Ada Junior High School
Ada, Oklahoma

Venable, Virginia
Chillicothe Junior High School
Chillicothe, Missouri

Vickers, Lori
Lake Braddock Secondary School
Springfield, Virginia

Vickers, Vanessa
Kings Glen School
Springfield, Virginia

Villanueva, Rene
John C. Martinez Junior High School
Parlier, California

Villasenor, Jose
Dana Middle School
San Pedro, California

Ward, Kimberly
Desert Horizon Elementary School
Phoenix, Arizona

Weeks, Josanna
Bellmont Middle School
Decatur, Indiana

West, Tyrel
Wheatland Junior High School
Wheatland, Wyoming

Whipple, Mike
Canandaigua Middle School
Canandaigua, New York

White, Schaefer
Richmond Middle School
Hanover, New Hampshire

Wilhelm, Paula
Wheatland Junior High School
Wheatland, Wyoming

Williams, Bonnie
Washburn School
Cincinnati, Ohio

Williams, Jason
Parkway West Middle School
Chesterfield, Missouri

Wiseman, Kristin
Glen Park Elementary School
New Berlin, Wisconsin

Wiseman, Megan
Glen Park Elementary School
New Berlin, Wisconsin

Yu, Veronica
Piñon Mesa Middle School
Victorville, California

Zipse, Elizabeth
Redlands Middle School
Grand Junction, Colorado

Acknowledgments (continued)

Emma Greig
"Spring" by Emma Greig, student. Reprinted by permission of the author.

HarperCollins Publishers
"Sarah Cynthia Sylvia Stout Would Not Take the Garbage Out" from *Where the Sidewalk Ends* by Shel Silverstein. Copyright © 1974 by Evil Eye Music, Inc. "I Saw What I Saw" by Judie Angell, from *Within Reach: Ten Stories*, edited by Donald R. Gallo. Copyright © 1995 by Judie Angell. Reprinted by permission of HarperCollins Publishers.

Henry Holt and Company, Inc.
"Stopping by Woods on a Snowy Evening" from *The Poetry of Robert Frost*, edited by Edward Connery Lathem. Copyright 1951 by Robert Frost. Copyright 1923 © 1969 by Henry Holt and Company, Inc. "The Judgment of the Wind" from *The Fire on the Mountain* by Harold Courlander and Wolf Leslau. Copyright 1950 by Henry Holt and Company, Inc. Copyright © 1978 by Harold Courlander and Wolf Leslau. Preface copyright © 1995 by Harold Courlander. Reprinted by permission of Henry Holt and Company, Inc.

Japan Foreign-Rights Centre on behalf of Shinichi Hoshi, and Stanleigh H. Jones, Jr.
"He-y, Come On Ou-t!" by Shinichi Hoshi, Copyright © 1978 by Shinichi Hoshi, translated by Stanleigh Jones. Reprinted by permission of Japan Foreign-Rights Centre and Stanleigh H. Jones, Jr.

Barbara S. Kouts, Literary Agent
"Birdfoot's Grandpa" from *Entering Onondaga* by Joseph Bruchac. Copyright © 1975 by Joseph Bruchac. Reprinted by permission of Barbara S. Kouts for Joseph Bruchac.

Little, Brown and Company
"Justin Lebo" from *It's Our World, Too!* by Phillip Hoose. Copyright © 1993 by Phillip Hoose. Reprinted by permission of Little, Brown and Company.

Merlyn's Pen, Inc.
"Grandpa's Hand" by Juli Peterson first appeared in *Short Takes: Brief Personal Narratives and Other Works by American Teen Writers*. Reprinted by permission of Merlyn's Pen, Inc.

William Morris Agency, Inc., and Fountain Pen, Inc.
"A Christmas Carol: Scrooge and Marley" by Israel Horovitz, an adaptation of Charles Dicken's *A Christmas Carol*, copyright © 1994 by Fountain Pen, Inc. Reprinted by permission of William Morris Agency, Inc., and Fountain Pen, Inc.

New Directions Publishing Corporation
"An Easy Decision" by Kenneth Patchen, from *The Collected Poems of Kenneth Patchen*. Copyright © 1949, 1957 by New Directions Publishing Corporation. Reprinted by permission of New Directions Publishing Corporation.

Reader's Digest Association, Inc.
"The Shadowland of Dreams" by Alex Haley is reprinted with permission from the August 1991 Reader's Digest. Copyright © 1991 by The Reader's Digest Association, Inc.

Linda Spisak
"Coming Out of the Storm" by Summer Spisak, published in *Magnetism '93*, a publication of the Humanities Magnet Program, Miami, Florida. Reprinted by permission of Linda Spisak.

Teaching Tolerance
"The Leader in the Mirror" by Pat Mora, from Fall '94 edition of *Teaching Tolerance*. Reprinted by permission of *Teaching Tolerance*, © 1994 Southern Poverty Law Center.

Rosemary A. Thurber
"The Princess and the Tin Box" from *The Beast In Me and Other Animals* by James Thurber. Copyright 1928, 1929, 1930, 1931, 1932, 1933, 1934, 1935, 1936, 1937, 1940, 1943, 1944, 1945, 1946, 1947, 1948 by James Thurber. Reprinted by permission of Rosemary A. Thurber.

Note: Every effort has been made to locate the copyright owner of material reprinted in this book. Omissions brought to our attention will be corrected in subsequent printings.

Photo and Fine Art Credits

Boldface numbers refer to the page on which the art is found.

H-cover: *Asphalt Dream*, Helen Kim, The Scholastic Art & Writing Awards; **Hv:** *Untitled*, Guevera Soliman, Walt Whitman High School, Bethesda, Maryland; **Hvi:** *Three Birds*, Judit Santak, from Rainforest for the Children: 1995 Calendar. Paintbrush Diplomacy, Courtesy of the International Children's Art Museum; **Hvii:** *Untitled*, Robert Wall, Overton High School, Memphis, TN; **Hviii:** (background) Dr. E.R. Degginger; (center) Peter Timmermans/Tony Stone Images; (bl) Kjell B Sandved/Photo Researchers, Inc.; (br) Courtesy of the author; **Hix:** (background) Brian Yarvin/Photo Researchers, Inc.; (center) Prentice Hall; (bottom) T. Wiewandt/Photo Edit; **Hx:** *Untitled*, ©1996 Robert Vickrey/Licensed by VAGA, New York NY; **H4:** (tl) *Portrait Of A Young Woman, c. 1470*, Piero del Pollaiuolo, tempera on wood. H. 19-1/4 in W. 13-7/8 in. (48.9 x 35.2 cm), Metropolitan Museum of Art Copyright © 1979/95 by the Metropolitan Museum of Art, Bequest of Edward S. Harkness, 1950. (50.135.3); **H5:** (top) *The Dunstable Swan made by a London goldsmith, c.1400.*, Copyright British Museum; (bottom) James Thurber/The Granger Collection, New York; **H7:** *Untitled*, Guevera Soliman, Walt Whitman High School, Bethesda, Maryland; **H8:** (background) Dr. E.R. Degginger; (bl) Michael Newman/Photo Edit; **H11:** Michael Newman/Photo Edit; **H13:** G.R. Roberts/Omni-Photo Communications, Inc.; **H14:** (top) Renee Lynn/Photo Researchers, Inc.; (bottom) Clarion Books; **H17:** Illustration from "Where the Sidewalk Ends" © 1974 by Evil Eye Music, Inc. Used by permssion of HarperCollins Publishers; **H18:** (left) Illustration from "Where the Sidewalk Ends" © 1974 by Evil Eye Music, Inc. Used by permssion of HarperCollins Publishers; (right) Michael Ochs Archives; **H20:** George/Archive Photos; **H21:** Bonnie Kamin/Photo Edit; **H22–23:** (background) Blair Seitz/Photo Researchers, Inc.; (center) Deborah Davis/Photo Edit; **H23:** The Bettmann Archive; **H24–25:** (background) Bonnie Kamin/Photo Edit; **H25:** (bottom) Bonnie Kamin/Photo Edit; **H26–27:** Chronis Jons/Tony Stone Images; **H28:** Orchard Books; **H30:** The Bettmann Archive; **H31:** *Studio Interior, 1917*, Stuart Davis, oil on canvas, 18-7/8 in. W. 23 in. Copyright © 1995 by the Metropolitan Museum of Art, George A. Hearn Fund, 1994. (1994.412); **H32:** Jerry Leff Assoc., Inc.; **H33:** The Bettmann Archive; **H35:** *Untitled*, Guevera Soliman, Walt Whitman High School, Bethesda, Maryland; **H37:** Prentice Hall; **H38:** (bottom) Peter S. Thacher/Photo Researchers, Inc; **H38–39:** (background) Victor Englebert/Photo Researchers, Inc.; **H40:** (left) Courtesy of the author, Photo by Herbert Cohen; (right) Courtesy of the arthor, Photo by Jaques Maquet; **H40–41:** (background) Herman Emmet/Photo Researchers, Inc.; (br) Giraudon/Art Resource, NY; **H43:** (background) Dale E. Boyer/Photo Researchers, Inc.; (br) Giraudon/Art Resource, NY; **H44:** Giraudon/Art Resource, NY; **H45:** Dr. E.R. Degginger; **H47:** *Three Birds*, Judit Santak, from Rainforest for the Children: 1995 Calendar. Paintbrush Diplomacy, Courtesy of the International Children's Art Museum; **H52:** Courtesy of the author; **H54:** (bl) Kjell B.Sandved/Photo Researchers, Inc.; **H54–55:** (background) Dr. E.R. Degginger; (center) Peter Timmermans/Tony Stone Images; **H55:** (bottom) Courtesy of the author.; **H56:** (left) Prentice Hall; (bottom) T.Wiewandt/Photo Edit; **H56–57:** (background) Brian Yarvin/Photo Researchers, Inc.; **H58–59:** (background) Robert Tang/Eskom International; **H60–61:** (background) Leen Van Der Slik/Animals, Animals; **H62–63:** (background) Robert Tang/Eskom International; **H64–65:** (background) Joseph VanWormer/Photo Researchers, Inc.; **H66–67:** (background) Robert Tang/Eskom International; **H69:** Bill Bachmann/New England Stock Photo; **H70:** Alan Oddie/Photo Edit; **H71:** Photo by Diane Lebo, Little, Brown and Company; **H72:** David Young-Wolff/Photo Edit; **H73:** Courtesy of Richard Connelly; **H75:** *Three Birds*, Judit Santak, from Rainforest for the Children: 1995 Calendar. Paintbrush Diplomacy, Courtesy of the International Children's Art Museum; **H77:** Harper Collins; **H80:** John Carroll Lynch as Marley in the Guthrie Theater's 1994 production of *A Christmas Carol* adapted by Barbara Field. Photo credit: Michal Daniel; **H83:** Charles Janasz as Bob Cratchit in the Guthrie Theater's 1992 production of *A Christmas Carol* adapted by Barbara Field. Photo credit: Michal Daniel; **H86:** Bob Davis as Bob Cratchit and Nathaniel Fuller in the Guthrie Theater's 1994 production of *A Christmas Carol* adapted by Barbara Field. Photo credit: Michal Daniel; **H90:** John Carroll Lynch as Marley and Richard Ooms as Ebenezer Scrooge in the Guthrie Theater's 1994 production of *A Christmas Carol* adapted by

Commissioned Illustrations

H140, H141: S.I. International (Artists' Representative)

Electronic Page Makeup

Larry Rosenthal, Tom Tedesco, Dawn Annunziata, Penny Baker, Betsy Bostwick, Maude Davis, Paul DelSignore, Irene Ehrmann, Jacob Farah, Alison Grabow, Gregory Harrison, Jr., Marnie Ingman, Laura Maggio, Lynn Mandarino, David Rosenthal, Mitchell Rosenthal, Rasul Sharif, Scott Steinhardt

Administrative Services

Diane Gerard

Photo Research Service

Omni-Photo Communications, Inc.